Laughing at My Alcohol Addiction

Hanging Out Without Drinking

By Benny N. Tran

ISBN:978-1-959376-30-9

Printed in the United States

Visit our Amazon author page to explore more books by Benny N. Tran. Follow for updates on new releases.

Scan for more Books

This book is for informational purposes only. It is not a substitute for professional medical advice, diagnosis, or treatment. Always seek the advice of a qualified health provider with any questions regarding a medical condition or before making changes to your health routine.

If you enjoy this book,
please give us a review.
We would really appreciate it.

INTRODUCTION

I used to think alcohol made life fun. Happy hour was my escape hatch, the party-starting elixir that unlocked something in me I didn't know existed—confidence, fearlessness, a looseness that felt essential in a world built on sharp corners.

At least, that's how it seemed, until the hangovers began to last longer than the good times, and the stories I laughed about started to sound tired—even to me. I thought I was choosing freedom every time I raised a bottle. Still, eventually, it became evident that I'd wandered into the opposite—a meticulously disguised trap, lined with laughter and "cheers," but padded with anxiety, regret, and self-doubt.

If you're anything like me, you won't realize you've crossed a line until you're looking back at it, blurry-eyed and wondering when fun turned into obligation. In my twenties, I drank because everyone did. At weddings, work events, family gatherings—there was always a reason, always someone urging, "Come on, just one more." Social norms, peer pressure, and the myth that drinking was essential for human connection wove themselves into my daily routine. At first, I told myself that I "deserved" to unwind. But slowly, choices faded into habits. Habits into cravings. Until it wasn't so much about celebration anymore; it was simply a part of my identity.

I wish I could say there was one dramatic rock-bottom moment—a DUI, a bar fight, some pivotal catastrophe—that snapped me awake. Instead, it was a slow slide: headaches I couldn't shake, mornings clouded by anxiety, and an ever-present tension just beneath my skin. Physically, I started getting sick more often. My sleep was restless, my energy dismal, my motivation shot. Emotionally, simple tasks felt daunting, and my temper frayed over minor annoyances. More than once, I woke up in a random location and couldn't remember how I got there. Yet I never thought I even had a problem with drinking. Without fail, Friday night rolled around, and the cycle repeated itself.

Eventually, the mirror became impossible to avoid—not just the literal one. It reflected the story I'd been telling myself: that I needed alcohol to belong, that I wasn't funny, interesting, or brave enough on my own. That drinking was normal, even healthy, as long as I could keep up.

One night, I realized something was off. My body didn't feel right, and minor health issues kept cropping up—I couldn't put my finger on what was happening, but I knew it wasn't normal. My stomach was in pain, and I was sick more often than not, and the drinks I once thought were harmless now seemed to be taking a toll. That's when it hit me: this wasn't just a habit anymore. My health was warning me, and I couldn't ignore it. Fun had turned into something that slowly wore me down, and it was time to take control.

Here's the wildest part: Saying goodbye to alcohol didn't make me lose my sense of humor, my friends, or my social life. If anything, I gained them back—this time, for real. The first few sober nights out were awkward, sure. I fumbled through those initial conversations, babysitting my water bottle like a nanny while everyone else cheered with a shot glass. I braced for questions, for skepticism. People notice when you break tradition, especially one wrapped in culture, romance, and friendship. But most of the time, I stayed strong because my health was on the line. And soon, what stood out wasn't my drink, but my presence —more alert, more engaged, and to my surprise, having more genuine fun.

The myths are powerful: Alcohol is essential to relax, to connect, to celebrate. Without it, you're missing out. But the joke is how dull and repetitive those nights had become, once I saw them clearly. I realized that alcohol wasn't unlocking my best self; it was making me dumb. Laughter is sharper now, memories stick, and mornings don't feel like punishment for the night before.

Hangovers signal your body's desperate protest against a substance it was never designed to process in large quantities. Sustained drinking does far more than sap your energy; it chips away at well-being, amplifies anxiety, disrupts sleep, and erodes genuine happiness.

You'll find plenty of science throughout this book: stories of what alcohol actually does to the body and brain, why it hooks us, and most importantly, how sobriety can transform your mind, mood, and relationships. I've explored the research and lived much of it myself.

But facts only take us so far. The journey away from drinking, for most people, isn't a neat line or a checklist of steps to follow. It's messy, personal, frustrating, and often hilarious in hindsight. You'll see echoes of your own experience in these pages —moments of temptation, flashes of doubt, unexpected triumphs, and tiny victories that add up over time.

I'm not here to judge or shame. If you love beer with dinner, or taking a shot with friends, that's your call. But if you've ever wondered whether alcohol is adding to your life—or quietly taking something away—you're in the right place. Maybe you've tried to cut back before, only to get pulled back in by tradition, expectations, or the sheer inertia of habit. Perhaps you suspect that deep down there's another version of you waiting under the buzz —a bolder, brighter person who doesn't need a drink to loosen up or fit in.

That's who you're about to meet. This book isn't a lecture or a demand—it's more like a hand extended across the bar, inviting you to the other side. I'll share my journey, what I've learned, and the strategies that helped me navigate cravings, peer pressure, and social situations without alcohol. Along the way, we'll question some of the assumptions and clichés that kept me stuck— including the idea that quitting means giving up all the fun.

The rewards go far beyond better mornings. When alcohol stopped occupying center stage, I noticed a spectrum of benefits that no one talks about: more profound sleep, steadier moods, clearer thinking, and a sharp uptick in self-respect. Relationships improved, not just because I remembered conversations, but because I was finally fully present. Saying no got easier, self-doubt quieter. Most unexpectedly, my sense of humor came roaring back—not forced or sloppy, but natural and unfiltered. The world seemed less threatening, and my capacity to handle its ups and downs grew stronger every week.

This isn't a promise that every day will be easy, or that you'll suddenly become a superhuman version of yourself. But I can tell you what you stand to gain: a clear mind, a body that's healing, and a sense of possibility that goes way beyond whatever you left behind in the bottle. You'll learn how to navigate parties, holidays, weddings, and even bar scenes—without feeling like you're missing out. You'll pick up skills for handling peer pressure and saying no, building authentic connections, and gently steering away when a drink is offered. Best of all, you'll discover a new perspective on fun—one that comes without regret, apology, or hazy memories.

So, welcome—no gratitude necessary. Let's raise a glass of water to discovering what happens when you ditch the old narrative and start writing your own.

Chapter 1: The Truth About Alcohol

Alcohol is often seen as just a simple way to unwind or socialize —a drink after work, a toast at a party, or a casual nightcap. Most people think its effects stop once the buzz fades or the hangover passes. But what if the impact of alcohol reaches far beyond these moments? What if it quietly shapes your mood, influences your decisions, and affects your relationships in ways you don't even notice?

Framing the Problem

A relaxing drink at the end of a tough week seems harmless. You might pour a glass of wine or crack open a beer, thinking it will melt away stress. The next day, though, everything feels off. Your mind is foggy. That easy feeling from the evening before turns into snapping at loved ones over small things or fighting an undercurrent of anxiety you can't explain. This is a reality check: alcohol doesn't just "take the edge off." It shapes how you feel, think, and act in ways that go far beyond what most people expect.

Ask a group of friends what comes to mind when they hear "alcohol harms," and most will mention the liver or drinking and driving. That's not wrong, but it barely scratches the surface. Alcohol slips into all corners of daily life. It changes moods, shifts priorities, and rewires relationships, sometimes so gently that you only notice in hindsight. A joke about needing a drink to unwind isn't just banter; it hints at how alcohol becomes woven into handling stress, loneliness, or boredom. Someone else might notice how get-togethers revolve around bars or breweries. These patterns feel ordinary, even comforting, until you stop and see what's really happening beneath the surface.

Beliefs about drinking often sound like rules that no one wrote down. "It's fine as long as I don't get drunk," or "I only drink socially, so it's not a problem." Some promise themselves— maybe after an awkward conversation or a bad headache—that quitting or cutting back would be easy. Most adults don't picture themselves in the stories of "problem drinkers." Yet this line between harmless and harmful isn't always obvious. Your brain and body react to alcohol even if you're counting your drinks or your hangovers feel mild. The way alcohol changes stress, happiness, and even sleep can slip past conscious awareness.

Everyday moments make these effects clear. There's the friend who gets loud and cracks jokes after a drink, then turns quiet and irritable the following day. Another might promise themselves they'll only have one but end up reaching for a second as their group orders another round.

The swinging door between calm and edge, social warmth and withdrawal, is one of alcohol's most reliable tricks. You don't have to drink to blackout or fight with friends to feel these effects. Even light, regular drinking—just a glass or two—turns restful sleep into fragmented tossing and turning. You wake up tired, less patient, less focused at work or at home.

Socially, alcohol creates invisible circles. A drinking get-together after work seems like a harmless chance to bond. But patterns emerge. Invitations, celebrations, and even comfort with certain people hinge on whether a drink is involved. Sometimes it becomes awkward to meet up without alcohol in the picture. Over time, these routines nudge alcohol from being an occasional treat to something at the center of relationships, shaping intimacy, routines, and even self-image. If drinks are a "reward," or a way to show up for friends, it gets harder to imagine social time without it.

Alcohol's influence grows quietly. Small changes build up: trouble getting up in the morning, sharper words with loved ones, feeling flat even when nothing is wrong. It's easy to chalk these up to work pressure or bad sleep. The real reason might be a slow adjustment inside your body. The liver starts to work harder. The gut feels unsettled. Nights that used to lead to deep sleep now leave you thirsty, waking up, or wrestling with headaches before your alarm.

The Physical Toll

Alcohol's path through the body starts within minutes of the first drink. The brain catches the effects right away, and that's when the symptoms of drinking start appearing. People often notice a warming or relaxing sensation, but this is the body being forced to work overtime. Take hangovers, for example. They aren't just "feeling rough." The brain's tissues actually swell a little because alcohol dehydrates the body and leads to inflammation. That's where pounding headaches come from: actual swelling and pressure in the brain. At the same time, alcohol flushes electrolytes like sodium and potassium out of balance, which triggers muscle cramps, feelings of weakness, and those waves of nausea. Even blood sugar swings get worse after drinking, thanks to alcohol's ability to block the liver from keeping energy levels steady. Many people find themselves sweaty, dizzy, or shaky the next morning. This is the body struggling to reset itself after being thrown off balance. What feels like a bad morning is actually your body running emergency repairs on damage it never asked for.

Alcohol also alters sleep from the very first night. While it may seem to help with falling asleep, it actually blocks REM sleep —the stage where the brain processes memories, dreams, and emotions. Research shows REM sleep can drop by up to 65% after just two or three drinks. At the same time, deep, restorative sleep declines. People wake more often during the night, and overall sleep quality drops sharply. Even moderate drinking can reduce deep sleep by 9–14%, leaving people tired, foggy, and unfocused —even after going to bed early.

Over time, the physical toll snowballs. The liver, which filters out toxins, cannot keep up with constant alcohol intake. At first, the liver builds up fat in and around its cells, which happens in up to 90% of people who regularly drink more than two or three drinks daily for a few years. This fatty stage often goes unnoticed. If drinking continues at this pace, a person will usually develop hepatitis, an inflamed, swollen liver that hurts and just doesn't work right. Up to 35% of regular drinkers will reach this stage at some point. After years, the final stage sets in: hard, scarred tissue —called cirrhosis—where the liver can't repair itself. This stage occurs in about 10-20% of those with ongoing heavy drinking. The effects are apparent in daily life: sluggishness, yellowed eyes or skin, and constant stomach upset.

Beyond the liver, alcohol puts pressure on the heart by weakening its muscles. Over months of repeated use—even just a few drinks every day—the heart starts to lose its strength to pump blood. People tire more easily, feel short of breath on stairs, and sometimes even notice swelling in their legs and ankles. Research shows rates of heart muscle damage are nearly doubled among moderate-to-heavy drinkers compared to those who abstain.

The digestive system also gets inflamed. The esophagus and stomach are lined with sensitive membranes that react to alcohol, leading to pain, heartburn, and sometimes open sores (ulcers). Up to 15% of regular drinkers will develop some form of digestive inflammation after five to ten years of steady alcohol use. Problems with diarrhea, indigestion, and even bleeding can appear.

Alcohol also throws the immune system out of rhythm. The body's natural defense against infections and illness is dulled, starting after just a few high-alcohol nights per month. People might notice that minor cold symptoms linger or simple wounds take longer to heal. Research reports that people who drink more than seven drinks per week are up to 30% more likely to catch respiratory illnesses than those who drink less or not at all.

One reality is that even "moderate" drinking, like two drinks almost every night, piles up fast. In half a year, that's over 350 drinks. Each round interrupts cells' ability to repair the tiny daily wear-and-tear, especially in places like the liver, stomach lining, and blood vessel walls. Over time, this adds up: sleep disruptions don't fully recover, organ tissues work harder, and the body gets stuck in a low-energy cycle.

These physical changes trigger a chain reaction. As brain inflammation, poor sleep, and constant repair demands accumulate, concentration drops and mood swings intensify. Exhaustion and imbalance blur together.

Mental and Emotional Health

Alcohol's effects on the body go beyond what you feel physically. When you drink, your brain chemistry shifts. These shifts kick off mood swings, impulsive decisions, and long-lasting anxiety. You might notice these changes after just a drink or two, long before you actually feel "drunk." Alcohol blocks certain messages between brain cells, lowering your ability to think clearly or control emotions. It also disrupts how your body manages hydration and sleep, setting you up for a chain of mental and emotional effects that stick around long after the hangover fades.

When you take that first drink, you may feel happier or more outgoing. Alcohol increases dopamine, the chemical that fuels short bursts of excitement and pleasure. You laugh louder, talk more, and worries shrink for an hour or so. But alcohol also slashes levels of serotonin and other mood regulators, which brings emotional shakeups later.

The cheerful high slides into irritability, stress, or even sadness once your body finishes processing the alcohol. This new low can kick in a few hours after drinking and last up to 72 hours. Some people snap at friends. Some get weepy or feel empty at work the next day. In real-time, these mood swings show up during parties too—one minute everyone is giggling together, and the next someone storms off or picks a fight. Many underestimate just how much alcohol can stir up mood changes, because the shifts can sneak up and blend into your routine.

Alcohol also triggers anxiety by changing how your nerves talk to each other. If your heart pounds in your chest after drinking, that's your brain trying to rebalance itself. During drinking, you might feel calm or fearless, but as soon as blood alcohol drops, anxiety comes roaring back. This starts because your brain slows itself down when alcohol is present, then rebounds by firing up stress hormones to overcompensate once the buzz fades. That's why you can feel jittery, panicked, or restless the morning after. This cycle repeats every time you drink: first a false sense of relaxation, then a spike in anxiety and worry. If you already struggle with anxiety or depression, this hit is often harder. Alcohol worsens existing symptoms by interfering with both sleep quality and hydration, pushing your mood further down.

The pattern shows up everywhere. Someone drinks on Friday night to unwind after a hard week. By Saturday morning, they wake with a racing heart and uneasy thoughts already spiraling. This anxiety can last for a full day or longer, leaving them fragile the next time something stressful pops up. And, for people with depression, these chemical swings create a steeper drop from the artificial high. It can feel like being trapped under a heavy cloud, where motivation and hope disappear for days.

Decision-making takes a big hit, even early into a night out. Your brain's risk filter slows down after a single drink because alcohol dampens the signals in the prefrontal cortex—the part that weighs long-term consequences. You may grab your keys thinking you feel fine but aren't safe to drive. Small choices, like sending a late-night text you regret, ordering more drinks than planned, or making risky bets, become common. After just two or three drinks, your ability to predict risks falls off a cliff. Some people start arguing or share secrets. Others agree to things they wouldn't do sober, then beat themselves up with regret the next day.

That relaxed feeling isn't all it seems. Alcohol blocks anxiety in the moment by dulling both stress signals and clear thinking. You pause, breathe out, and it feels like your worries fade away. This effect is temporary and artificial. As alcohol leaves your system, your stress response rebounds twice as hard. The brain boosts stress hormone production to get back to normal, but often overshoots, adding tension and worry for hours or days. Using alcohol for stress management is like borrowing happiness from tomorrow.

It's easy for alcohol to slip into the background of daily life. Going to a get-together or happy hour may seem harmless, but attending becomes an unspoken expectation. If someone skips the drink, their colleagues might ask if everything's okay, making the absence of alcohol stand out more than its presence. During family weddings, the champagne toast often gets more attention than the speeches. Birthday parties sometimes show friends giggling over a bottle of liquor as the ultimate symbol of fun, or lonely characters solving heartache with a stiff drink. On social media, filtered images of Hennessy bottle at sunset or craft beers at Friday gatherings gain plenty of likes, nudging people to share their own moments with alcohol as the centerpiece. Over time, these signals tell everyone that drinking is not just allowed—it's expected. Anyone who resists can feel like an outsider in their own community.

Drinking goes beyond parties—it can shape personal relationships too. Some couples only seem to connect when alcohol is involved. I've dated people who loved drinking so much that giving it up felt like risking the relationship itself. Staying home or doing something healthy together seemed dull to them; their happiest moments were tied to a glass in hand, surrounded by others drinking. The sad truth is, I met many of these partners through drinking. Quitting alcohol meant letting go not just of the habit, but of an entire social world built around it.

These expectations aren't made up. Research shows that alcohol is woven into every social layer, from families who light up a dinner with a bottle of wine, to neighborhoods where weekend beer gardens fill up faster than local parks. The more someone sees alcohol as "normal," the harder it is to question whether it's healthy or necessary.

Media and marketing add to this pressure. Ads show glamorous parties, attractive people laughing with cocktails, and stressed parents relaxing "responsibly" with a glass of something strong. Even responsible drinking campaigns can backfire, attaching the idea of fun and relaxation to alcohol while urging moderation. Over years, these images become blueprints for how to act, what to expect, and how to treat drinking as a sign of maturity.

Showing up at an event where everyone's drinking and you're the only one sober instantly makes you stand out. You'll get asked the same question twenty or thirty times that night—"Why aren't you drinking?"—like you've broken some unspoken rule. People glance your way as if you don't belong there, a party pooper in a room full of laughter. When everyone's buzzed and lost in their own world, you're stuck on the outside looking in. And if you're introverted or shy, that sense of not fitting in hits even harder.

Another familiar story centers on moderation. People like to say, "A little won't hurt—some even say it's healthy." "Just one" sounds harmless, even virtuous. But in my experience, very few stop there. One becomes two, then three, until moderation is no longer a boundary but an idea. Science is unforgiving here: even moderate drinking raises risks for certain cancers and liver disease, with effects that build quietly over time. Choosing water, seltzer, or a night alcohol-free sets a different example—one that celebrates the moment without the hidden cost. The best nights are the ones you actually remember.

Willpower myths trap a lot of people trying to cut down or quit drinking. Many like to say, "If I really wanted to, I could stop anytime." The first few days might go smoothly, but soon social events, stress, and routine temptations start breaking that resolve. Alcohol has a way of working itself into daily life so quietly that willpower alone isn't enough to fight it. What actually helps is structure—having a plan, a support network, and new habits that make drinking less appealing. Trying harder isn't the answer; trying smarter is.

Cultural cues are everywhere, but they don't have to control the story. Myths can lose their hold when people see through the rituals and discover routines, rewards, and ways to feel good— without putting alcohol at the center.

Reference List

Hytner, S., Josselin, D., Belin, D., & Bowden Jones, O. (2024, December 24). *Myths and facts about alcohol use disorder: a Delphi consensus study.* Brain Communications. https://doi.org/10.1093/braincomms/fcaf035

Sudhinaraset, M., Wigglesworth, C., & Takeuchi, D. T. (2016). *Social and Cultural Contexts of Alcohol Use: Influences in a Social-Ecological Framework.* Alcohol Research: Current Reviews. https://pubmed.ncbi.nlm.nih.gov/27159810/

Chapter 2:How Alcohol Affects Your Brain and Body

Have you ever noticed how a single drink can change the way you feel—making you more relaxed, more talkative, or maybe even a little clumsy? Have you wondered why that shift happens, or what's really going on inside your body when alcohol takes effect? Maybe you've brushed off those moments of forgetfulness or sudden mood swings as nothing serious. But what if those quick changes are just the surface of something deeper—something quietly reshaping how your brain and body work over time? Let take a look beneath the surface to uncover how alcohol interacts with your biology, altering your mood, memory, and behavior in ways that can linger long after the glass is empty.

Why Biology Matters

Those weekend drinks with friends might be secretly rewiring your brain. That might sound dramatic, but every sip of alcohol you take changes the way your brain and body function. Alcohol isn't just a regular beverage or a simple way to relax after a long week. It's a psychoactive substance—a type of chemical that travels through your bloodstream, crosses into your brain, and disrupts the signals that help you think, feel, and move. Even a single glass of wine or a cold beer can shift your mood, slow your reflexes, and dim your judgment, often before you feel noticeably different.

Alcohol acts fast, and the changes aren't always apparent at first. Think about the feeling of being just a little tipsy at a party. You might laugh more easily, talk louder, or lose track of time. That's alcohol affecting your brain's ability to manage impulses and decisions. Ever fumble your keys on the way home or misread someone's tone during a conversation? Alcohol can throw off your coordination and twist your understanding of social cues, sometimes with consequences you may not remember clearly the next day. Those minor misjudgments might be harmless for some — but for others they can spiral into arrests, or hospital visits.

You can feel this shutdown happening even when you think you're fine. For me, sleepiness was more than just a drowsy side effect—it was total shutdown. I lost count of how many times I passed out in my car after a night of drinking. I'd start the engine, thinking I'd rest my eyes for a split second, then wake up to a dead car battery and needing to call friends and family for assistance.

Emotional changes build on top of these shifts in brain chemistry. Maybe you've noticed yourself laughing harder, feeling braver, or getting mad after a few drinks. That's alcohol chipping away at your brain's ability to regulate mood. Emotions can swing quickly as natural self-control slips away. Some people might feel relaxed and at ease, while others become aggressive or anxious. These mood swings are part of why alcohol sometimes leads to decisions you'd never make if you were sober. The same neurotransmitters influencing thought also shape how you react emotionally, making the effects impossible to separate.

If you think making bad choices while drunk is harmless, let me tell you about my friend Hao. His group of friends was known for getting into fights in the bar scene I used to hang around. To them, fighting after a few drinks was just normal—they had low impulse control. But their recklessness didn't stop at strangers; sometimes they turned on each other. It might sound ridiculous, but that's how alcohol twists judgment and amplifies emotions. It's all fun until one night goes too far. Hao's younger brother has been in prison for nearly fifteen years for manslaughter. One night, at a Korean karaoke bar in California, he was extremely drunk and got into a heated argument with another man over a girl. In the chaos, he went to his car in the parking lot and pulled out a gun, thinking it wasn't loaded, just to scare him. It was loaded. One impulsive decision, one second of blurred thinking, and a man's life was gone—and another's forever changed.

Brain Chemistry and Addiction Pathways

Alcohol works directly on the central nervous system, acting as a psychoactive substance that changes the way the brain functions. This process starts from the very first sip, where alcohol begins interacting with crucial brain chemicals called neurotransmitters. These are the messengers that allow brain cells to communicate, and when alcohol enters the system, it alters the delicate balance between them.

The first major player is GABA, a neurotransmitter that slows down brain activity. Think of GABA as a car's brake system. When you drink alcohol, it boosts GABA's effects. More GABA means an even greater slowing down of messages in the brain, similar to pressing the brake pedal harder. This creates that familiar sensation of relaxation and calm, but it can also bring on drowsiness and clumsiness. People may stumble or slur their words, not because they intend to, but because their brain's usual control over movement and speech has become less responsive.

At the same time, alcohol lowers glutamate activity. Glutamate is usually like the gas pedal, helping you think sharply and store new memories. When alcohol dampens glutamate, the result is mental confusion and forgetfulness. This is why even after just a few drinks, remembering details like where you parked your car, or what someone just told you, becomes a challenge. Missing appointments, repeating stories, or losing track of time are common signs that alcohol has disrupted simple memory circuits.

This explains a lot of moments I've lived through myself. There were nights when I'd leave the bar, confident I could handle the drive, only to realize miles later that I was heading the wrong way. Once, I drove forty minutes in the opposite direction of home, too drunk and exhausted to think clearly. I could feel my body shutting down, my eyelids heavy, my mind foggy. If I hadn't pulled over, I probably wouldn't have made it. I ended up parked in a stranger's driveway, sleeping it off in my car. By some miracle, I woke up early and drove home—before the homeowners noticed and called the cops.

Then there was my friend T-Bone. He was the kind of drinker who'd blackout and lose control completely. When he got drunk, his temper came out—he'd start swinging at his own friends, slurring insults, completely unaware of what he was doing. Most of the time he'd miss, stumble, or knock himself out against a wall. It was chaotic, almost comical at first, until the damage started to show. Over the years, people began to distance themselves from him, including me. Alcohol didn't just make him forget nights—it cost him relationships that took years to build.

Alcohol also cranks up dopamine, the brain's main reward chemical. Dopamine works like a volume knob for pleasure. When you drink, dopamine surges, making you feel good and encouraging you to keep drinking. This boost gives alcohol its addictive potential. The more often you drink, the more your brain learns to crave that dopamine rush. Over time, the brain starts to prioritize alcohol over everyday rewards, reinforcing the cycle of drinking even when you know it can have negative consequences.

This cocktail of changes affects how you make decisions. When GABA is high and glutamate is low, clear thinking and careful judgment are replaced by impulsivity. Everyday scenarios make this obvious. Imagine someone at a party who suddenly decides to buy an expensive round of shots for everyone, or promise something they can't deliver the next day. These impulsive choices seem great in the moment, but alcohol has blunted the brain circuits that usually help weigh risks and consequences. This can also show up in riskier behaviors, like driving after drinking or picking fights with strangers you'd normally walk away from. It also gives you a false confidence, making you take risky actions that can endanger your life.

Memory and learning abilities are also hit hard. Repeated alcohol use disrupts the hippocampus, a region of the brain responsible for forming new memories. Simple tasks, like following a conversation or learning a new skill, become much more difficult. That's why people under the influence sometimes wake up the next day unable to remember major parts of their night.

With repeated alcohol use, deeper changes occur, creating physical dependence. The brain tries to adjust to the constant presence of alcohol by reducing its own natural GABA activity and increasing glutamate to compensate. This creates a new normal in the brain, where alcohol is needed just to feel steady. If someone stops drinking suddenly, they may feel shaky, anxious, or irritable—signs of withdrawal caused by the brain scrambling to rebalance itself.

Over time, these changes ripple outward into mood, behavior, and relationships. A brain wired for alcohol rewards may lead you to act in ways you wouldn't otherwise choose, showing up in emotional swings, difficulty connecting with others, and a stronger pull toward situations that keep feeding the cycle. The brain's changing chemistry never works in isolation, pushing shifts in how you feel, think, and behave long after the last drink.

Emotional and Behavioral Effects

Impaired judgment means the usual "pause and think" step before acting gets skipped, leading to risky choices: hookups with strangers, sleeping at completely strangers' home. One night out can shift from laughter to regret fast. I've seen it myself—people convinced they're fine to drive home end up calling me the next day to bail them out of jail, facing community service, DUI classes, and huge fines. It's a brutal wake-up call that a few drinks can destroy far more than just your night.

These emotional and behavioral effects trace directly to what alcohol does in the brain. As alcohol boosts GABA and dopamine, it makes us feel good while silencing the natural warning systems that keep us from reckless actions. At the same time, alcohol suppresses another neurotransmitter, glutamate, which normally helps us think clearly and respond to situations thoughtfully. The chemical crash as alcohol wears off can bring irritability, sadness, or anxiety—the classic "hangxiety" that follows a heavy night. This biological tug-of-war—feeling high, then low—shows up in behavior: joy, recklessness, regret. It's the same cycle every time.

Physical Effects on the Body

Alcohol's path through the body starts with its impact on the liver. Early signs of liver trouble appear within just a few weeks of heavy drinking. A person might notice tiredness, tenderness on the right side below the ribs, or unexplained digestive upset. Inside the liver, fat starts building up in cells—this condition is called fatty liver and can develop in as little as two weeks of regular, heavy drinking. Blood tests show rising levels of ALT and AST enzymes, which doctors use as markers for liver stress. If drinking continues, the next stage is alcoholic hepatitis, bringing symptoms like jaundice, fever, and abdominal pain within a few months to several years of repeated abuse. Long term, up to about 15% of heavy drinkers develop cirrhosis over ten to twenty years; here, scar tissue replaces healthy cells, making the liver hard and shrunken.

Beyond the liver, alcohol's chemical effects ripple into the heart and blood vessels. Drinking causes a temporary widening of blood vessels, giving a flushed appearance and a feeling of warmth. While this may seem harmless, repeated episodes— especially from daily or binge drinking—can lead to elevated blood pressure. Hypertension may develop within just a few months of heavy alcohol use, significantly increasing the risk of stroke and heart attack.

Alcohol also disrupts the heart's rhythm. A person may notice a racing heartbeat or skipped beats—known as arrhythmia— within hours of drinking. Over time, chronic alcohol use can weaken the heart muscle, resulting in cardiomyopathy, a condition where the heart struggles to pump blood efficiently. Symptoms often include shortness of breath, swelling in the legs, and fatigue, sometimes appearing after only a few years of heavy drinking.

These cardiovascular issues not only reduce stamina for everyday activities but also heighten vulnerability to sudden events like stroke. For instance, consuming just one drink per day raises stroke risk by approximately 5%, and heavier drinking patterns push that risk even higher.

Moving through the digestive system, alcohol irritates and inflames the sensitive lining of the stomach almost immediately. After a night of drinking, a burning pain in the upper abdomen signals gastritis, a warning that the stomach lining is already inflamed. Continued drinking breaks down the layer protecting the stomach, letting stomach acid create open sores, or ulcers. These can appear within months, causing persistent pain, nausea, and even bleeding. Alcohol also inflames the pancreas. Acute pancreatitis may bring sudden, severe abdominal pain and vomiting after a few days or weeks of heavy drinking. If drinking continues, this can shift into chronic pancreatitis, leaving the pancreas scarred and unable to make valuable digestive enzymes or regulate blood sugar. People with chronic pancreatitis often develop diabetes, lose weight unexpectedly, and feel weak after meals.

Alcohol reaches the immune system through a web of chemical changes. Just a single episode of heavy drinking can reduce the number of white blood cells for up to 24 hours, leaving people more open to viral and bacterial infections. Chronic drinkers catch illnesses like pneumonia or tuberculosis twice as often as those who drink little or none. Recovery from infections also takes longer; for instance, healing from severe colds or flu stretches on average 2-4 days longer for heavy drinkers. Alcohol makes vaccines less effective and slows wound healing, further raising the risk of complications from everyday sicknesses.

Disrupted sleep is another key effect. Alcohol sedates the brain at first, but later in the night it disrupts REM sleep—the deep stage where learning and memory strengthen. People who drink before bed fall asleep quickly, but wake up throughout the night, feeling unrefreshed in the morning. Lack of REM leaves them struggling with focus and memory, leading to brain fog. This fog shows up as trouble following conversations, making decisions, or remembering details at work or school. Chronic sleep disruption has ripple effects—reaction times slow, mistakes increase, and the chance of accidents rises. These impacts are clear after just a few days of late-night drinking, but long-term sleep disruption raises risks for conditions like depression and anxiety.

Each body system interacts with the next. Liver damage leads to higher toxins in the blood, which can worsen heart rhythm problems or affect the ability to fight infections. Sleep problems cause fatigue, slowing healing from illness and sapping the energy needed to recover from organ stress. Early warning signs like stomach pain after drinking, tiredness, or frequent sickness are calls for attention. Some forms of damage, like fatty liver, can start to heal with weeks of sobriety. Others, like scarred liver or chronic heart problems, may last for life, but catching these changes early can help reverse some effects and protect future health.

Long-Term Consequences

Alcohol travels to every organ in the body, but the brain changes shape and function the most. Imaging studies reveal a shrunken cortex—the wrinkled outer layer of the brain—especially in people with years of drinking behind them. Over time, the volume of gray matter, which processes information and helps with decision-making, memory, and self-control, shrinks up to 1.6 times faster in heavy drinkers than in others. The prefrontal cortex, critical for planning and impulse control, becomes thinner and less active. The hippocampus, a memory control center, often loses up to 10% of its volume in severe alcohol users. This means recalling new information or even the events of last night can become almost impossible.

Cerebellum shrinkage is also common, leading to gait disturbances and worsened balance, sometimes mistaken for early signs of aging but actually due to alcohol's toxic effect. Alcohol blocks the growth of new brain cells, especially in the hippocampus and cortex, accelerating neurological wear and tear. People sometimes compare these effects to the slow shrinkage of a sponge left out in the sun—it dries out, and little by little, loses its structure and flexibility.

Long-term alcohol use also cuts levels of serotonin and dopamine, two neurotransmitters vital for mood and motivation. After enough exposure, natural serotonin and dopamine production drop, leaving people feeling joyless, tired, and unmotivated unless drinking again. These losses are part of the reason heavy drinkers face a risk of dementia up to three times higher than nondrinkers, with clear links between continued drinking and memory loss, confusion, and even full-blown Wernicke-Korsakoff syndrome—a severe brain disorder most often found in people with chronic alcoholism.

Many times, after a day of heavy drinking I found myself lying in bed all day feeling hopeless. That sense of despair took over and consumed my entire day. My productivity collapsed, and as I got older it only got worse—it took multiple days to recover. I asked myself: Why am I doing this to myself? Such a waste of time and energy, chasing something that destroys my health and gives no real benefit. I only ever felt "happy" again when I kept drinking, and that only led to more addiction—a spiral of hopelessness that made things worse.

Emotional health gets tangled in this web of chemical chaos. Feeling down or worried prompts some to drink, but alcohol actually worsens depression and anxiety over time. Drinking changes cortisol levels, the hormone responsible for stress, so the brain expects alcohol to calm it whenever problems arise. This creates a feedback loop: someone feels stressed, drinks to calm down, but the next day stress returns worse than before. The relationship between alcohol and depression becomes self-feeding; low mood and fatigue linger even with small breaks from drinking. Real-world signs include irritability, trouble sleeping, and swings between anger and sadness for no clear reason.

Alcohol also rewires the emotional reward system. Each drink delivers a jolt of dopamine, making the brain crave more. Over months or years, the brain expects to only feel pleasure when drinking, pushing everyday joys—like time with friends or a good meal—into the background. This explains why heavy drinkers may lose interest in work, hobbies, or relationships, a condition doctors call anhedonia.

The cumulative effect of these brain, mood, heart, liver, and immune changes leaves a person less resilient, older than their years, and at high risk for life-shortening diseases. Each step along this path is visible in day-to-day struggles with memory, focus, energy, and physical well-being—every outcome stacking on top of the last, turning what begins as occasional use into a cascade of permanent harm.

Reference List

Iranpour, A., & Nakhaee, N. (2019, April 1). *A Review of* Alcohol-*Related Harms: A Recent Update*. Addiction & Health. https://doi.org/10.22122/ahj.v11i2.225

Mann, R. E., Smart, R. G., & Govoni, R. (2003). The Epidemiology of Alcoholic Liver Disease. *Alcohol Research & Health*, *27*(3), 209. pmc.ncbi.nlm.nih.gov/articles/PMC6668879/

Chapter 3: The Gut Factor

Even a single heavy drinking session can irritate the gut lining. The intestinal barrier, a layer of cells that normally keeps toxins and bacteria contained, becomes more permeable under the influence of alcohol. When this protective barrier weakens, bacterial products can leak into the bloodstream, triggering inflammation throughout the body. Over time, repeated exposure compounds the damage, leaving the gut more susceptible to infections, digestive issues, and nutrient malabsorption.

Alcohol also disrupts the balance of gut bacteria. Beneficial microbes decline while harmful bacteria increase, a shift known as dysbiosis. This imbalance affects digestion, immune response, and even brain function. Signals from the gut communicate with the brain through the gut–brain axis, influencing mood, cravings, and cognitive clarity. The result is a feedback loop: alcohol harms the gut, the gut signals the brain, and cravings or anxiety can intensify, making moderation more difficult.

The combination of leaky gut and dysbiosis creates systemic stress. Inflammatory compounds released from the gut can reach the liver, heart, and other organs. This worsens the very issues alcohol initiates elsewhere. This hidden pathway explains why some effects of drinking—fatigue, brain fog, low mood—persist even after the alcohol itself has left the system. It's not just the amount consumed; it's the ongoing disruption to a critical internal ecosystem.

Disruptions in the gut don't always produce obvious signs at first. Some early indicators include bloating, irregular bowel movements, and mild stomach discomfort. Fatigue, brain fog, and even changes in mood can appear before any digestive pain is noticeable. These subtle symptoms reflect the body's response to inflammation and microbial imbalance, signaling that the gut is under stress long before serious illness develops.

Over time, chronic alcohol use compounds these effects. Nutrient absorption decreases as the gut lining becomes inflamed and less efficient. Vitamins and minerals critical for energy, immunity, and brain function—such as B vitamins, magnesium, and zinc—may be depleted. This combination can create a cycle where fatigue and cognitive decline push someone toward continued drinking, further damaging the gut and prolonging recovery.

Supporting gut recovery doesn't require extremes, just consistent care. A diet rich in fiber, fermented foods, and plenty of water helps restore beneficial bacteria and strengthens the intestinal lining. Avoiding additional irritants like excessive processed sugar or alcohol allows the gut to stabilize more quickly.

Sleep and stress management also play a role in recovery. The gut communicates constantly with the brain, so improving sleep quality and reducing stress helps rebalance the gut–brain axis. Over time these steps restore energy, mental clarity, and digestive regularity, allowing your body to heal from the strain alcohol imposed.

Natural Remedy for The Gut

Even after stopping alcohol, the gut needs support to fully recover. The intestinal lining and microbial community take time to repair, and targeted natural remedies can accelerate this process. Certain foods, herbs, and lifestyle practices help reduce inflammation, restore beneficial bacteria, and strengthen the gut barrier. This gives the body a better foundation for overall health.

Several natural foods and herbs can help the gut recover after alcohol:

Probiotics

Probiotics are live microorganisms that support a healthy balance of gut bacteria. They can be consumed through fermented foods like yogurt, kefir, kimchi, and sauerkraut, or as supplements. Once in the gut these beneficial bacteria help restore microbial diversity disrupted by alcohol, strengthen the intestinal lining, and reduce inflammation. Scientific studies show that probiotics improve digestion, support immune function, and communicate with the brain through the gut–brain axis. This helps stabilize mood and cravings while repairing gut damage.

Milk Thistle

Milk thistle contains silymarin, a powerful antioxidant compound that protects liver cells from alcohol-induced damage and supports liver regeneration. Taking milk thistle as a supplement or tea helps reduce inflammation, prevent scarring, and enhance the liver's natural detoxification processes. Research shows that silymarin strengthens liver function, improves enzyme levels, and accelerates recovery in people with alcohol-related liver damage.

Polyphenol-rich Foods

Polyphenols are compounds found in foods such as berries, green tea, dark chocolate, and pomegranate. They act as antioxidants in the gut protecting cells from oxidative stress caused by alcohol-induced inflammation. Polyphenols feed beneficial bacteria, suppress harmful species, and promote a more diverse microbiome. Research indicates that these compounds can improve the intestinal barrier, reduce systemic inflammation, and even support cognitive function through gut-brain signaling. Including these foods regularly strengthens the gut's resilience and accelerates recovery after heavy drinking.

Ginger

Ginger contains bioactive compounds, primarily gingerol, that have anti-inflammatory and antioxidant properties. Drinking ginger tea, adding fresh ginger to meals, or taking supplements helps soothe the stomach lining and reduce nausea. Scientific studies show ginger modulates inflammatory pathways in the gut, reducing damage to the intestinal barrier and improving digestive function. By calming inflammation and protecting gut cells, ginger supports the repair process after alcohol has disrupted the microbiome.

Turmeric (Curcumin)

Turmeric's active compound curcumin is well-known for its anti-inflammatory effects. It can be consumed as a spice in cooking, in golden milk, or as a supplement (ideally with black pepper to enhance absorption). Curcumin helps reduce gut inflammation, strengthen the intestinal lining, and support the growth of beneficial bacteria. Research shows it decreases gut permeability — protecting against leaky gut — and helps restore a balanced microbiome after alcohol-related stress. Regular use supports both digestive and systemic recovery.

Bone broth

Bone broth is made by simmering animal bones and connective tissue for an extended period. This releases collagen, amino acids like glycine and proline, and minerals. Consuming a cup of bone broth daily helps repair and maintain the gut lining, reduce inflammation, and improve nutrient absorption. Studies indicate that these compounds strengthen the intestinal barrier and support immune function, helping the gut recover more efficiently after alcohol-induced damage.

Hydration

Adequate water intake is essential for gut function. Drinking enough water helps flush bacterial toxins, maintain the mucosal lining of the intestines, and support nutrient transport. Even mild dehydration can slow the repair of gut cells and reduce the efficiency of digestion. Scientific evidence shows that proper hydration assists in maintaining gut barrier integrity, aiding recovery from inflammation and alcohol-induced stress.

Reference List

National Institute on Alcohol Abuse and Alcoholism. (2014). Single episode of binge drinking linked to gut leakage and immune system effects. National Institutes of Health.https://www.niaaa.nih.gov/news-events/news-releases/single-episode-binge-drinking-linked-gut-leakage-and-immune-system-effects

Alcohol or Gut Microbiota: Who Is the Guilty? (2019). Microbiome. https://pubmed.ncbi.nlm.nih.gov/31540133/

Chapter 4: The Hidden Costs of Drinking

"You were stuck with how much again at the bar?" my friend Nancy asked, half laughing, half shocked. I told her about another night gone wrong—a story that had become a pattern among drinkers. I always complained that drinking was expensive and that the people I met in those places rarely brought any real value into my life. Bars attract all kinds: freeloaders who vanish when the bill arrives, groups who drink on someone else's tab, and the bad drunks who start fights and drag you into their chaos. Every night felt like a repeat—money wasted, time lost, and energy drained on people and situations that went nowhere.

It's not just about the money. Alcohol brings out the worst in people—creeps, troublemakers, and those who lose all sense of boundaries. I've seen decent women go home with complete strangers, and I've heard plenty of horror stories from waitresses working in these environments. Some talk about seeing men slip something into a woman's drink while everyone else is too distracted to care.

Before you know it, you're surrounded by people running from their problems, not solving them. It's not about judging anyone—there are good people in every community—but they're the exception, not the rule.

Financial Impact

A night out for me used to cost around $400 back then. In today's prices, with inflation, that same night would easily reach double. The group I hung out with loved drinking Hennessy at first, but over time they kept switching to pricier bottles—first Cordon Bleu, then Don Julio 1942, which goes for top dollar in most Vietnamese hostess bars. These bars aren't cheap: food, mixers, and tips add up fast. Some guys hand-tip the girls directly, hoping to get lucky, and the ballers hand-tip up to $100.

If you've never been to a Vietnamese-style hostess bar, it's basically a karaoke lounge where waitresses—usually attractive women—sit, talk, and drink with customers. They get paid commissions on bottle sales, so the more you drink, the more they earn. It's a clever trap. I still remember my first time stepping into one when I was 21, turning 22. Back then, these places were known for fights, shootings, and easy hookups. Some of the waitresses even worked as escorts to make extra cash.

Over time, the scene got worse and more expensive. What started as a karaoke bar with flirtatious hostesses evolved into lap-dance bars charging $50 per lap-dance, double what it used to be. Eventually, many turned into underground clubs run by thugs, with shootings happening every few months. It was a complete money pit. I didn't realize how deep I was getting until it became routine—and by then, all my friends were part of that world, making it even harder to walk away.

There were other spots I liked going to—clubs, downtown lounges, Korean bars, KTVs, even country music bars—but no matter where I went, they were all expensive. If you're a drinker living that party lifestyle, you know drinking is rarely ever cheap. And if you want to show off, play the big boss, or look like the cool one in the group, the bill climbs even faster.

If you think a night out drinking is expensive, wait till you get unlucky and catch a DUI like me or many of my friends. The fines are brutal, spending a night in jail is humiliating, and those court-ordered weekend trash pickups are a pain. Add mandatory DUI classes on top of it, and the costs—both money and time—pile up fast. Some of my friends never learned their lesson, racking up second and even third DUIs.

I still remember one guy from DUI class bragging about having close to ten DUIs—and he was only in his early thirties. A girl in class called him out, thinking he was lying, but the instructor just nodded and said, "He's telling the truth. I've seen him in here plenty of times." The guy laughed and said, "I might be young, but I'm a high achiever." Everyone chuckled, knowing all they could do at that point was laugh off their mistakes.

In my opinion, health expenses are one of the most brutal parts of being an alcoholic. The body takes hits that money can't always fix—and whatever can be repaired comes with a heavy price tag. Alcohol damages nearly every organ, and recovery costs pile up fast.

There are real stories of alcohol poisoning that end in tragedy, leaving families with funeral costs they never expected. I once heard about a young woman named Cindy—a wife and mother of two—who drank herself to sleep one night and never woke up. My friend Julie drank so much that she ended up in the emergency room, needing IV fluids to treat dehydration and alcohol toxicity.

Another friend, Howie, passed out drunk on a curb, fell forward, and broke both of his front teeth. The dental repair alone cost him a fortune. I've had my share of medical visits too—constant stomach pain sent me to the doctor several times, and I've seen plenty of others deal with ulcers from drinking on an empty stomach or never giving their body a chance to heal.

Alcohol's real price doesn't just hit your wallet—it drains your health, your time, and sometimes your future. You can replace money, but you can't replace the parts of yourself it slowly destroys.

Relationships and Social Life

Sitting across from me is a person I find highly attractive. I ask her to take a shot with me, and she seems happy to join. We're both drunk, hitting it off, exchanging numbers — the night couldn't get any better. We go home our separate ways.

The next morning, I text her. No reply. A few days later, she texts back saying she just saw my message. We have a few good conversations over text, but it's always inconsistent — off and on, like she's half there. I finally ask her to hang out, and when the day comes, silence again. I start making excuses for her in my head — "Maybe she was in an accident, maybe she forgot." Then she finally replies, saying she went out drinking and was too hungover to move. We reschedule. It happens again.

Excuse after excuse. Eventually, I'd had enough. I stopped reaching out, and she didn't seem to care. I thought maybe something was wrong with me, but years later I realized it wasn't me at all — it was the kind of people I kept meeting in those environments. The drinking scene attracts unreliable people, people who live for chaos and instant gratification. Even my own friends were the same — showing up late, flaking without notice, or ditching me for another party. For a long time, I thought that's just how people were. Only later did I learn that it wasn't society — it was the alcohol culture.

I started to question my friendships. Did people care about me, or were they just drinking buddies—connections built on shots and nonsense rather than anything real? Maybe they stuck around because I was always the one paying. I covered most of the tabs back then, but I didn't care; I thought my success made it worth it.

I met people constantly, and sometimes I'd go home with them, thinking I was making real connections. But looking back, I realize most of it was just drunken impulse, not genuine attraction or understanding. None of it lasted beyond the bar. Most of the people I met, we never went on a proper date—our version of a "date" was sitting across from each at a bar. Over time, my idea of what was normal started to blur. I wasn't around sober people, so I didn't even know what normal was anymore.

This cycle is exhausting. Each round of conflict chips away at what trust remains. Hurtful words said under the influence can't be unsaid—no matter how many times "sorry" is repeated later. Family bonds fray, friendships crack, couples drift apart.

Career and Productivity Loss

One thing I've noticed among my friends is how low their productivity really is. I always ended up paying for drinks because most of the people around me weren't making good money. They jumped in and out of jobs, unable to hold one for long or move up. When you're constantly calling in sick because you're too hungover to work, you're not going to keep that job for long. It gets even worse when you get a DUI and lose your license. A few of my friends kept driving anyway, taking huge risks just to get by. Living in constant survival mode like that is dangerous—and exhausting.

Looking back, I can say with confidence that I'd be far better off if I hadn't spent all my money at bars. I had almost no savings because every paycheck went straight into drinking. The only people making real money were the bar owners. Everyone around me was in the same or worse situation—even the high earners. They'd show off at the bar, drive luxury cars, and then go home to live with their parents because they never saved a dime.

The people hit hardest were the waitresses working in those bars. They drank with customers every night, always a little buzzed or worse. Ten years later, I'd see them still there—same bar, same routine—but now worn down from years of alcohol and stress. Their income depended on staying attractive and entertaining customers, but time and drinking took their toll. The late nights, the constant partying, and the lifestyle aged them faster than they ever expected.

It didn't just take a toll on the waitresses—it trapped them, just like the rest of us. They never really learned any new or transferable skills to help them escape the bar scene and find a better job. Their whole career became centered around drinking and serving drinks. As newer, younger girls showed up and started taking away part of their tip income, they found themselves in a worse position every year, with nowhere else to go.

The saddest part is seeing new faces enter the scene every year, replacing the ones who burned out before them—repeating the same cycle of addiction and self-destruction. You watch it happen over and over, and eventually you realize the scene doesn't just chew people up—it replaces them without a second thought.

The Erosion of Clarity

You ever run into that one friend you've known for years who's always at the bar, acting up? The same person who starts the night calm and happy, but two hours in, they're slurring their words, getting angry, and yelling at strangers. You feel trapped—you don't want to get pulled into their drama, but you can't just leave them to get arrested or hurt. I've had plenty of those nights, worrying about friends like that while barely holding my own drinking in check.

They say alcohol kills brain cells, and I believe it. One of my close friends, Cutsaw, told me he never used to black out when he drank, but as he got older, his mind just isn't the same. Now he'll be in the middle of a conversation and suddenly wake up not remembering how he got home alive. It happens more and more often. If you've ever watched a group of drunk people while sober, you can literally see the decline—slow reactions, sloppy speech, no sense of control. The more they drink, the more their brains deteriorate.

My friend Alison would always end up crying when she drank, emotions spilling out every single time. Another friend started turning violent, taking out his anger on his wife. I had to distance myself from him before it got worse. Watching people lose themselves like that—mentally, emotionally, morally—is what made me start questioning this lifestyle.

The hidden impact of alcohol is like a shot of fruity soju — sweet, smooth, and easy to drink. You don't feel drunk at first, so you keep going. Slowly, it creeps into your daily life, touching every part of it. Before you know it, you're a different person, but you don't even realize when the change happened. You start blaming bad luck or circumstances, never suspecting the real cause. That's how alcohol works — quietly, gradually — until one day your life is a drunk mess, and you can't remember where it all started.

Reference List

CDC. (2024, August 6). *Data on Excessive Alcohol Use*. Alcohol Use. www.cdc.gov/alcohol/excessive-drinking-data/index.html

Kulak, J., Heavey, S., Marsack, L., & Leonard, K. (2025, February). *Alcohol Misuse, Marital Functioning and Marital Instability: An Evidence-Based* Review *on Intimate Partner Violence, Marital Satisfaction and Divorce*. Substance Abuse and Rehabilitation; Informa UK Limited. doi.org/10.2147/sar.s462382

Sacks, J. J., Gonzales, K. R., Bouchery, E. E., Tomedi, L. E., & Brewer, R. D. (2015, November). *2010 National and State Costs of Excessive Alcohol Consumption*. American Journal of Preventive Medicine. doi.org/10.1016/j.amepre.2015.05.031

Chapter 5:My Turning Point

More than half of adults who struggle with alcohol say it takes a serious wake-up call—an event that shakes them to their core—to realize change is necessary. For some it's a health scare. For others, a broken relationship or lost opportunity.

My turning point came after years of ignoring the signs. One night, I went drinking like usual and came home violently sick, vomiting far more than normal. At that point, binge drinking was part of my routine—throwing up was just something that happened. I told myself I was fine because I looked young for my age and went to the gym almost every day. But none of that protected me from what was going on inside.

A few days later, I took a break from drinking, thinking I just needed to rest. When I finally grabbed a beer again, a sharp pain shot through my stomach—the worst pain I'd ever felt from alcohol. I thought maybe I'd developed a stomach ulcer like some of my friends had. Still, I didn't go to the doctor. I waited another week, then another month, testing myself each time with a few sips. Each time, the same searing pain came back instantly. That's when I knew something was seriously wrong. My body was warning me that I'd crossed a line, and if I didn't stop, there might not be another chance to turn things around.

Choosing Change

During this period of change, I realized I could no longer drink—maybe not ever again. That thought alone was terrifying. My mind flooded with questions: "Is my life over now? How will I ever enjoy anything again if drinking was all I knew?" For years, alcohol had been part of my identity. Now, without it, I felt lost. Friends kept calling, trying to drag me back to the bars, tempting me to "just come out for a bit." But deep down, I knew I couldn't. I needed to rest and figure out what came next. If alcohol was no longer part of my life, I had to find something new to live for.

I asked myself what I truly enjoyed outside of drinking—what actually made me feel alive. I'd always loved sports and staying active, so I decided to rebuild my life around that. I spent more time at the gym, joined a yoga class, signed up for a hiking group, MMA training, and even a Ninja Warrior-style fitness program. Those choices didn't just change how I spent my time—they changed how I saw life itself.

Finding New Purpose

I started to meet new people from all my gym classes and fitness activities. They were different—healthy, stable, and sober. We could actually have intelligent conversations instead of the usual drunk nonsense. My biggest fear about quitting drinking was losing my social life. I used to think, "How will I ever meet new people or date again without alcohol?" But I was meeting better people—people who had control of their lives, not emotional wrecks pretending to have fun.

For the first time, I started enjoying life without drinking, and it honestly shocked me. My emotions became steady; I wasn't angry or moody for no reason anymore. My thinking cleared up, and my decisions made sense again. I felt normal—more than I had in years. All my classes together cost about $500 a month, which might sound like a lot, but that used to be one night at the bar. It was the best trade I ever made.

Finding Stability

After being off alcohol for a while, my emotions started to stabilize. I wasn't getting angry over small things anymore, and I wasn't getting overly sensitive or offended at every little comment. I felt calmer. My mind saw things with more clarity. I argued less with friends—old and new—and I could actually have real conversations with people I dated because I wasn't emotionally all over the place. My mood felt steady for the first time in years. Even little frustrations didn't hit as hard. Life no longer revolved around alcohol and being drunk all the time.

I didn't realize how aggressive or intense I used to be until I stepped away from drinking. When you're in it, you convince yourself, "This is just how I am." But a lot of that "personality" was just alcohol messing with my emotions. Without it, I could finally see the parts of myself that needed work—and I could actually fix them.

The first time I went back to the bar sober, it was like watching my past self from the outside. I could hang out without drinking, stay in control, and speak clearly. Meanwhile, my friends were slurring, repeating themselves, and stumbling around. I felt embarrassed realizing I used to be exactly like that.

People think alcohol makes them more social, more confident, more attractive. But when you're sober and someone drunk comes up to talk to you—sloppy, off-balance, and talking nonsense—it's not charming. It's uncomfortable. It's messy. It's not confidence—it's desperation. And the only people who respond to that energy are others in the same spiral. No wonder the only relationships I formed in that lifestyle were with people who were also a hot mess.

I still went to the bars sometimes, but only to sit, eat, and talk. I turned down drinks every time, and trust me—people don't like when you break the drinking pattern. They'll push, joke, tease, and try to wear you down. But after a while, when they saw I wasn't budging, they stopped asking. Some respected it, others just gave up trying. Either way, the pressure faded.

Sitting there sober, I could see everything clearly for the first time. The loud arguments, the sloppy flirting, the fake confidence —it all looked different from the outside. I realized that used to be me, and I felt embarrassed just remembering it. The more I watched, the more disconnected I felt from that world. It didn't look fun anymore. It didn't look exciting. It just looked empty.

Chapter 6:Rebalance and Self-Actualization

The first few weeks after quitting alcohol can feel strangely quiet. Life slows down, but not in a peaceful way—more like a fog settling in. Things that once felt exciting now feel flat. Food doesn't taste as good, jokes don't hit the same, music doesn't move you like it used to. This is the hangover no one talks about —the dopamine crash that follows when your brain has spent years chasing chemical highs.

Alcohol floods the brain with dopamine, the chemical that fuels motivation, reward, and pleasure. It tricks you into believing you're happy, confident, and connected, but the cost is steep. Over time your brain stops producing its own dopamine at normal levels. So when you quit drinking, you don't just lose the buzz— you lose the ability to feel normal joy. That's why early recovery can feel like emotional numbness, a kind of gray period where nothing feels meaningful.

But this phase isn't permanent. It's the brain's way of rebuilding balance after years of being hijacked. Each sober day the dopamine system begins to reset. Natural pleasures begin to return—exercise, sunlight, a good meal, or real connection with others start to feel good again. The challenge is being patient— trusting the flatness will fade and genuine happiness will return naturally, just like before.

Slow and Steady Wins the Race

After being clean for a while, my dopamine levels started to balance out. Instead of dumping it all at once—feeling amazing for one night and miserable for the next few days—my brain began releasing dopamine in a smoother, more natural rhythm. Life became easier to enjoy. It wasn't about short bursts of euphoria anymore; it was about a steady sense of calm and happiness that felt real.

This taught me something important: chasing quick highs always comes with a crash. Having a little bit of good every day beats one night of fake joy followed by a week of feeling empty. When your brain learns to run on balance instead of extremes, even simple things—eating a meal, going for a walk, talking with someone you care about—begin to carry real weight again.

Eventually, I drank again, but only a little. A beer here, a shot there—never more. I stayed completely in control. I know most people are better off quitting entirely, and honestly, I probably should too. But for me, I reached a place where alcohol lost its power. When I did drink, it mostly gave me headaches. That's when it hit me—it was never the alcohol that made life fun. It was the people, the vibe, and the moments.

If you threw a New Year's party and gave everyone fake drinks that tasted real but had no alcohol, they'd still laugh, dance, and celebrate. The joy comes from connection, not the bottle. You don't have to be drunk to have fun—you just have to be present. Once I realized that, I stopped linking alcohol with happiness. I could cheer a bottle of water and still feel just as much joy as before—maybe even more.

Understanding what drives you to drink is only half the battle —the other half is having a plan for those moments. Matching each major trigger with a healthier response creates room for change. If work stress is a regular culprit, a quick breathing exercise or a walk around the block can offer a pause between feeling and action. If social situations are the trigger, practicing short sober conversations or planning to leave an event early helps break old patterns.

Battling boredom? Try making a list of simple, enjoyable options—reading, hitting the gym, cooking something new for dinner—so you aren't caught off guard. Relationship conflicts call for learning a few respectful communication tools so discussions don't always spiral into old escape routes.

A small shift in awareness can reveal how fast emotional triggers can pile up, leading to unpredictable moods or strong urges. That's where the real work begins: not just spotting triggers, but being ready for what comes next. Recognizing and mapping your own triggers is the groundwork for building consistent, reliable sober habits that last.

Early Sobriety Emotional Challenges

Going through early sobriety often feels like facing the world without armor. For years, you might have counted on a drink to turn down the volume on anger, sadness, or nerves. That liquid shortcut worked for a while—until it didn't. Alcohol is a maladaptive coping mechanism because it offers comfort in the moment but disrupts your ability to handle emotions naturally, leading you into a cycle that's hard to break.

Take irritability. Maybe you snap at your partner after a long day, or minor work setbacks leave you fuming. When drinking, your brain's stress response gets thrown off. Normally, when you get frustrated, your body releases stress hormones, and then your natural coping skills kick in to bring you back to baseline. With repeated alcohol use, your brain stops trusting those built-in tools and waits for alcohol to "reset" your system instead. Without that crutch, stress feels as if it's dialed up to eleven. Your body may ache, you tense up quickly, or find yourself clenching your jaw for no obvious reason. This physical discomfort is common in early sobriety, and it's a double whammy—your mind is on edge, and so is your body.

Sadness often hits harder in early sobriety, and there's a biological reason for it. Alcohol artificially boosts neurotransmitters like GABA and dopamine, creating a chemical sense of calm, pleasure, or emotional numbness. When drinking stops, those levels drop sharply. The brain that relied on alcohol to regulate mood is suddenly forced to function without its shortcut. Colors feel duller, laughter comes slower, and small disappointments feel heavier than they should. It's not weakness

—it's chemistry. After years of borrowing feel-good chemicals from alcohol, the brain is paying that debt back. This adjustment period can last weeks or even months, during which emotions feel sharper and less manageable. The key is understanding that this phase is temporary. Your brain isn't broken—it's relearning how to regulate mood on its own.

Anxiety is perhaps the most confusing of these emotional spikes. The nervous system that used to be slowed by regular drinks becomes hypersensitive once alcohol is removed. Your heart might race before a meeting, hands tremble at family gatherings, or your breath catches when checking your bank account. Withdrawal makes this worse by changing how your brain processes adrenaline and cortisol. It's like someone replaced your steady heartbeat with a hummingbird's—fast, fluttery, always ready to startle. This uptick in anxiety is not just in your head; it's rooted in the way alcohol reshaped the wires and signals of your nervous system.

Think about everyday stress—missing a deadline at work or getting bad news from family. When alcohol was available, those moments were quickly erased with a drink. Over time, the brain learns a dangerous lesson: discomfort doesn't need to be processed, only avoided. Each drink reinforces the habit of outsourcing stress relief instead of building internal coping skills. When alcohol is removed, those skipped skills are suddenly required—but they're underdeveloped. That's why early sobriety can feel overwhelming. You're not weaker; you're relearning emotional regulation that alcohol quietly replaced for years.

The real trap shows up when life throws a curveball—an unexpected bill, an awkward party where everyone else is drinking, or a fight with a friend. In those moments, old urges can surge without warning. The brain has been conditioned to associate alcohol with relief, so stress automatically triggers cravings, even when the conscious mind wants to stay sober. During early sobriety, emotional swings are common because the system that once muted discomfort is gone. Until the brain recalibrates its emotional baseline, reactions feel sharper, urges louder, and distress harder to ignore. Every feeling hits raw.

The timeline for emotional downturn varies. In the first days and weeks, reactions tend to be most intense as the body clears alcohol and the nervous system recalibrates. During this period, the urge for relief can surface in many forms—overeating, constant distraction, or even reenacting old drinking rituals. Over time, the brain begins restoring balance, though stress can still trigger strong emotional responses.

Understanding why these reactions feel so extreme helps reframe them as part of healing rather than personal failure. By facing irritability, sadness, or anxiety head-on—naming them instead of numbing them—you create space to build healthier responses. Gradually, you learn to trust your internal emotional thermostat again, adjusting to life with clarity and confidence rather than relying on old shortcuts. This is the real work of recovery, supported by both science and consistent daily effort.

Rebuilding Self-Confidence

Waking to that familiar dread after a night of drinking, the mind races with memories of promises left unkept—another sick-day call to work, unread messages from friends, the fading excitement for a family gathering. These everyday stumbles chip away at self-esteem one excuse at a time. Someone might promise not to drink before the big meeting, only to arrive late, flustered, or call in sick. Or say yes to a family dinner, but end up avoiding it, afraid of questions and judgment. Small lies to cover drinking, or anxiety-filled apologies after angry words, create guilt that lingers long after the headache is gone. Each of these moments stacks up, creating a story about failure and disappointment that weighs heavy on self-worth. Over time, people with alcohol dependence often blame themselves, thinking, "Why can't I just get it together?" These self-blaming cycles trap people, making it harder to picture any other life.

The good news is that every decision in early sobriety offers a way out of the cycle. Neuroscience shows that habits form when actions repeat over time and the brain's reward system rewires itself. Each time someone chooses not to drink, even in small ways, they strengthen the mental pathway that supports self-trust. Getting through a workday without calling in sick, sticking to a morning routine, or having an honest conversation with a friend without alcohol—these moments are building blocks for a new self-image.

A simple five-step routine, the "Trust-Building Blueprint," makes this growth visible. Start each evening by listing three small goals for tomorrow, such as eating breakfast, calling a supportive friend, or showing up on time for work. For each goal, write down a clear, concrete action that will make it happen. The next day, focus on doing what's on the list, then record which tasks were completed. Afterwards, reflect on what it felt like to follow through and notice how even checking off one task builds hope. Every step builds a sense that "I can count on myself," which is the core of self-esteem in recovery.

Tracking victories in a "Victory Journal" gives setbacks less power. At the end of each day, write down every win, even those that seem minor—like making it through a hard hour sober, going to bed early, or turning down an invitation to drink. When noting these wins, include physical and emotional states: did the muscles relax, did breathing slow, did thoughts feel calmer? If there was a tough moment or even a slip, jot down one thing learned that could help tomorrow. Sharing this progress with a friend, sponsor, or group every week builds connection and accountability, which protects self-worth over time.

Reference List

Justyna Zaorska, Małgorzata Rydzewska, Kopera, M., Paweł Wiśniewski, Trucco, E. M., Paweł Kobyliński, & Jakubczyk, A. (2023, May 12). *Distress tolerance and emotional regulation in individuals with alcohol use disorder.* Frontiers in Psychiatry; Frontiers Media. https://doi.org/10.3389/fpsyt.2023.1175654

Schick, M. R., Nalven, T., & Spillane, N. S. (2021, October 22). *Drinking to Fit in: The Effects of Drinking Motives and Self-Esteem on Alcohol Use among Female College Students.* Substance Use & Misuse.
https://doi.org/10.1080/10826084.2021.1990334

Chapter 7: The Real Gateway Drug

Growing up, I constantly heard warnings in commercials and school programs that marijuana was a "gateway drug"—the first step toward harder and more dangerous substances. That message was repeated so often that it felt unquestionable. As an adult, I see that the picture is far more complicated. What stands out to me now is not how marijuana supposedly opens the door to addiction, but how deeply alcohol is woven into everyday life around the world.

Alcohol is legal, socially accepted, and often encouraged in ways no other drug is. It is present at celebrations, business events, family gatherings, and even moments of stress or grief. In many places, it is sold in nearly every grocery store or corner shop, making it one of the most accessible psychoactive substances on the planet. Most people are exposed to alcohol long before they encounter any other drug, often during their teenage years or earlier.

What makes alcohol especially powerful is not just its availability, but what it teaches. It introduces the idea that altering your state of mind is a normal way to relax, cope, celebrate, or socialize. It lowers inhibitions, increases impulsivity, and places people in environments where risk-taking feels acceptable. Under the influence of alcohol, boundaries blur, judgment weakens, and decisions that might otherwise feel off-limits suddenly seem harmless or temporary. This is where alcohol quietly becomes a gateway—not necessarily because it causes drug use directly, but because it changes behavior, expectations, and tolerance for risk.

It's difficult to label marijuana as the primary gateway when alcohol reaches nearly everyone first. In many parts of the world, marijuana remains restricted, regulated, or illegal, while alcohol faces few meaningful barriers. Entire industries are built around encouraging people to drink more, not less. From advertising to social pressure, alcohol is framed as a reward, a solution, and a rite of passage. Avoiding it often requires a lot of effort.

<u>The Starting Point</u>

From what I've seen in my own life and around me, alcohol is often the starting point. It's the substance that normalizes intoxication, opens the door to poor decisions, and creates the conditions where other substances enter the picture. In that sense, alcohol isn't just another drug—it's the one most people are trained to underestimate. And for me, that makes it the most dangerous gateway of all.

I had been exposed to other substances before alcohol, but none of them crept into my life the way alcohol did. They came and went — I tried them and moved on. Alcohol blends into normal life—it's served with food, at graduation, at family events. It doesn't feel extreme. It feels ordinary. That's what makes it dangerous. You don't need to plan for it or cross a psychological line to start drinking. It's a small step that feels harmless, even responsible. But once you're drunk, decision-making collapses. Alcohol doesn't just lower inhibition—it rewires what feels acceptable in the moment.

With other drugs, I always backed out quickly. They felt like too big of a step, too intense, too obvious. Alcohol was different. It was gradual. One drink became several, and before I knew it, I was drunk and open to things I never would have tried sober. When someone passed a joint, it didn't feel like a major decision. I was already in the moment, already feeling good, already careless. So I said yes. That's how alcohol traps people—it turns "no" into "why not?" I saw this happen not just to me, but to many friends around me.

Marijuana is the lighter end of that slope. What came after was darker. In some Asian bars, it's common to see people smoking turbo outside. Turbo is crack cocaine rolled into a cigarette, and it was treated casually—almost like part of the nightlife. I never would have touched it sober. But drunk, surrounded by people doing it, offered again and again, it stopped feeling extreme. For a period of time, I used it. Alcohol had already stripped away my caution, and adding something stronger felt like just another small step, not a big leap.

It didn't just intensify the damage—it stacked it. My emotions were already unstable from drinking; adding crack made everything worse. I was lucky enough to stop before it went further. I watched others not get that chance. One older friend moved from turbo to smoking it through a pipe. Within months, he lost his job, his family, and his home. He ended up sleeping near creeks and railroad tracks with others who had followed the same path. Seeing that up close made one thing clear to me: alcohol wasn't just part of the problem—it was the doorway that made all of this possible.

When Alcohol Meets Cocaine

When you go out drinking, there's a pattern that becomes impossible to ignore. Groups suddenly drift off to the bathroom together. Someone taps their nose or flashes a key like a signal. They disappear into a stall or a quiet corner, away from eyes. If they're bold, they don't even bother hiding it. A small bag comes out, and everyone knows what's inside—cocaine. In recent years, these two substances have become closely linked. Bars, clubs, house parties—wherever heavy drinking happens, cocaine often follows. The overlap is hard to miss. Among drinkers, cocaine use is far more common than people like to admit, almost treated as a normal extension of the night. It's spoken about casually, passed around casually, and rarely questioned in the moment.

Alcohol plays a critical role in this pairing. Cocaine creates a false sense of alertness, tricking you into thinking you're less drunk than you are. This lets people keep drinking far longer than their body can handle — hours, sometimes days — without realizing how much damage they're doing. I've experienced this firsthand, with serious consequences, and I'm lucky to have come out of it alive. The cocaine boost feels like a second wind, but it's an illusion. Your body is still absorbing every drink, even if your brain can't feel it anymore. Some even believe it sobers them up enough to drive, a dangerous myth that has led to many deaths.

When cocaine is circulating, offers come easily. If you're drinking in that environment, chances are high you'll be offered some sooner or later—often multiple times in a single night.

For me, cocaine was never something I liked long-term. I value sleep, and cocaine destroys it. The jittery energy, racing thoughts, and empty crash afterward were a huge turn-off. But for a lot of people, it turns into something much worse—an extra addiction stacked on top of alcohol. Cocaine rarely stays on its own. It often becomes a doorway to harder stuff, including crack. I've watched people slide from casual use into something dark without even realizing how far they'd gone. A night that starts with a few drinks can quietly turn into losing your job, losing your family, and sleeping in a creek smoking crack.

From the Bars to the Creek

Story One: The Jolly Nurse

When I say "the creek," I mean the natural waterways that run through the city—often reinforced with concrete and connected to flood-control channels. In the city where I live, these areas have become common gathering places for homeless encampments, drug addicts that live off the grid. It's the kind of place where stories like Kathy begin."

I met my friend Kathy through the party scene—she was friends with my crew, and her ex-boyfriend went to high school with me. Kathy was a jolly, happy girl who loved going out drinking and always invited people over to her house. Somehow, what started as alcohol turned into smoking crack. The worst part was that her dad ended up smoking with her. Their addiction spiraled, and before long, Kathy and her father were selling crack just to fund their own addiction. They weren't discreet about it, which eventually led to a home robbery. That robbery turned into a gunfight between her dad and the intruder. Her father was shot but refused to go to the hospital and died a few days later.

After that, Kathy completely unraveled. She smoked even more and got involved with a man much older than her—around her father's age—who was also addicted to crack. They smoked together constantly. Over time, he took control of her life and began pimping her out to fund their habit. Before all of this, Kathy was a nurse, making good money, surrounded by people who cared about her. Her life was stable, full of laughter, and moving forward.

A few years later, I came across a YouTube video where someone was interviewing homeless people and sharing their stories. Kathy appeared in the video. She looked like she had aged fifteen years in a very short time. She was living in a tent near a creek, sleeping in a play area with a much older man. Watching that video felt unreal, knowing where she came from and how far she had fallen.

Story Two: A Second Chance Lost

Zane was always a troubled kid. He joined a gang at a young age and was already getting into serious trouble in his teens, eventually committing a hardcore shooting that landed him in prison for nine years. When I met him again after all those years, we caught up quickly and even went drinking together. He had a bad habit of being shady with money, so I started keeping my distance.

After he got out of prison, Zane seemed to turn his life around. He was working in the union and making excellent money, earning a pension and nearly $100 an hour on night shifts —an extreme amount, especially before COVID and inflation hit. He loved going to bars, and with his selfish nature, whenever someone offered free drugs, he was more than happy to take them.

A few months later, I saw him walking into our old bar we normally drank at, the Courtyard. At first, I didn't recognize him; he looked older, thin, and had a new hairstyle. Then I realized it was Zane. He had become homeless and was smoking crack nonstop. Crack had suppressed his appetite so much that he barely ate. He showed off his ripped six-pack from losing all the weight from his suppress appetite—but he looked like a skinny crack addict. In about six months since I distanced myself, he had gone from a high-paying union worker with a bright future to living on the streets, losing not only his job but also his soon-to-be wife, who broke off the engagement after discovering his addiction.

How fast drugs can ruin a person is insane. One night out, one series of choices, and everything he had worked for was gone —his job, his future wife, and his entire life trajectory.

Story Three: From Radiant to Unrecognizable

Anna was one of those girls everyone noticed in high school—confident, outgoing, and always surrounded by attention. After high school, she met her boyfriend who introduced her to drinking, and alcohol quickly became part of her everyday life. What started as casual nights out slowly shifted into something worse. Drinking led to smoking crack, and before long the two of them were spending nights in the creek. For many people deep in addiction, the creek becomes a gathering place. It's where users congregate, where supply is always available, and where dealers know they can reliably make money. Once someone starts spending time there, they're no longer just experimenting—they're fully inside that world.

When the relationship ended, Anna looked for another boyfriend to fill the same role. Another friend of mine was drawn in by her beauty, even though drugs were never his interest. She slowly pulled him into her world—drinking first, then crack, then nights spent chasing the next hit. She was still emotionally tied to her ex, and that lingering attachment may have been the only thing that saved my friend. He eventually broke up with her and, thankfully, snapped out of the trap. He managed to step away and rebuild his life. Anna didn't.

Her addiction deepened, and over the years she cycled in and out of jail on drug-related charges. After a long stretch inside, I didn't see her for a long time. When I finally did, it took me a moment to recognize her. I ran into her outside a supermarket, and the change was shocking. Her skin looked damaged and worn, her body exhausted, as if years had passed all at once. Crack had taken a visible toll—people who use it often become fixated on picking at their skin, sometimes for hours, and combined with poor nutrition and constant stress, it leaves lasting damage and accelerates aging.

She was with a new partner she met while incarcerated. In drug-heavy environments—especially jail and the streets—relationships often form around survival rather than attraction. Access to drugs, protection, or resources becomes leverage. Over time, those dynamics blur personal boundaries and reshape behavior in ways people never planned.

In addiction and incarceration, relationships stop being about genuine connection. They form around survival — who has drugs, who offers protection, who controls resources. People adapt to those environments in ways they never would have outside of them. Anna was no different. The longer she stayed in that world, the more her relationships were shaped by dependency and power rather than real choice.

This world is full of exploitation, and I've seen it more times than I wish I had. When addiction takes hold, desperation lowers defenses and people become vulnerable in ways they never imagined. Some individuals use drugs as a tool for control—offering shelter, protection, or substances in exchange for sex or obedience. It isn't talked about openly, but it happens.

The line from *Menace II Society*—"Can I suck your dick for some crack?"—wasn't fiction or exaggeration. I've heard real versions of that exchange, and what disturbed me most was not just that it happened, but that some people talked about it afterward with pride, as if exploiting another person at their lowest point was an accomplishment. Watching that made it painfully clear how far addiction can strip people of empathy, boundaries, and basic human decency in people.

Anna met her partner in prison, where these dynamics were already in place. Access to drugs became a form of control, and over time Anna adapted to survive within that structure. Addiction didn't just take her health or freedom—it reshaped her identity, her relationships, and her sense of self.

Alcohol can be an incredibly powerful gateway drug. One addiction can easily lead to another, eventually spiraling into a life of suffering. Environments shaped by this cycle rarely bring out the best in people—they magnify vulnerability, poor choices, and exploitation.

Reference List

Kirby, T., & Barry, A. E. (2012, August). Alcohol as a gateway drug: A study of US 12th graders. *Journal of School Health, 82*(8), 371–379. https://doi.org/10.1111/j.1746-1561.2012.00712.x

McCance-Katz, E. F., Kosten, T. R., & Jatlow, P. (1998). Concurrent use of cocaine and alcohol is more potent and potentially more toxic than use of either alone—A multiple-dose study. *Biological Psychiatry, 44*(4), 250-259. https://doi.org/10.1016/S0006-3223(97)00426-5

Kandel, D., Griffin, E., & Levine, A. (2017). *Columbia researchers study how alcohol influences cocaine addiction.* Columbia University Mailman School of Public Health.

Chapter 8: Overcoming Peer Pressure

Most of the pressure to drink never came from alcohol itself—it came from people. From someone I wanted to impress, and from social situations where saying no felt risky. In many Asian cultures, including Vietnamese culture, refusing a drink—especially from an older person or inside someone's home—can be seen as disrespectful. Alcohol becomes more than a drink; it becomes a signal of respect, harmony, and belonging. Saying no can feel like rejecting the person, not the alcohol.

What I learned is that peer pressure doesn't disappear—you get better at handling it. The more times you say no, the easier it becomes. You start finding your own ways to deflect, redirect, or shut it down without creating tension. It's like being pitched a product you don't want: at first you freeze, but over time you learn how to counter smoothly.

Understanding Peer Pressure

Peer pressure isn't just a social concept—it's a biological one. When adults are around others who are drinking, the brain's reward system becomes more active. Social approval, belonging, and acceptance trigger dopamine release in the same neural circuits involved in pleasure and motivation. In simple terms, fitting in feels good at a neurological level. This is why group behavior is contagious and why resisting it can feel uncomfortable even when no one is explicitly pressuring you. The brain quietly registers social alignment as a reward worth pursuing.

At the same time, alcohol weakens the very system responsible for resisting that pull. The prefrontal cortex—the part of the brain responsible for judgment, impulse control, and long-term decision-making—becomes less effective after even moderate drinking. While the reward system stays active, the brain's braking system softens. This imbalance makes it harder to say no, harder to slow down, and easier to justify "just one more," especially when others around you are doing the same. The decision feels social, but the mechanism is neurological.

Social environments also activate the brain's threat-detection system. The amygdala responds to potential rejection or exclusion as a form of risk, creating subtle anxiety when someone considers going against the group. In adults, this doesn't show up as fear—it shows up as discomfort, awkwardness, or the urge to comply. The brain treats social friction as something to avoid. Combined with alcohol's dampening effect on self-control, this explains why peer pressure doesn't disappear with age—it simply becomes quieter, more internal, and easier to rationalize.

The Brain Under Social Pressure

Peer pressure is not primarily a moral failure or a lack of willpower. It is a neurobiological response to social threat and reward. The adult brain constantly evaluates social environments for signals of safety, status, and belonging. When those signals shift, neural systems adjust behavior automatically, often before conscious reasoning catches up.

At the center of this process is the brain's reward circuitry. Social approval activates the same dopamine pathways involved in food, sex, and money. Acceptance is coded as reward; rejection is coded as loss. When an individual senses that agreement, imitation, or compliance will increase social reward—or prevent social loss—the brain biases decisions in that direction. This happens even when the person intellectually disagrees with the behavior. The calculation is not "Is this right?" but "Does this keep me inside the group?"

At the same time, perceived social exclusion activates threat systems. Cortisol levels rise, attention narrows, and risk tolerance changes. Under these conditions, people become more likely to conform, less likely to challenge authority or group norms, and more likely to adopt behaviors that signal alignment. This is not weakness; it is the brain prioritizing survival in a social species.

In adults, peer pressure rarely looks overt. It shows up as subtle shifts: changing opinions in meetings, mirroring group attitudes, tolerating behavior one would normally reject, or delaying action to avoid standing out. The mechanisms are quieter than in adolescence, but they are more deeply integrated into identity, career, and long-term social positioning. The brain is not reacting to peers as "friends," but as gatekeepers to resources, status, and stability.

This is why adult peer pressure is often more powerful than teenage peer pressure. It operates through systems tied to livelihood, reputation, and belonging—and it does so largely below conscious awareness.

Breaking the Pressure Loop

Peer pressure persists because it feeds on repetition. Each time a person conforms to reduce discomfort or gain approval, the brain learns that compliance works. Dopamine reinforces the behavior, stress decreases, and the neural pathway strengthens. Over time, this creates a loop: anticipate social tension, adjust behavior, receive relief. The longer the loop runs, the less conscious the decision becomes.

The key to disrupting this cycle is not resistance through force, but interruption through awareness and delay. When social pressure appears, even a brief pause allows higher-order cognitive systems—primarily the prefrontal cortex—to re-enter the decision process. This shifts behavior from automatic alignment to deliberate choice. The goal is not to oppose others, but to prevent the brain from defaulting to the fastest relief option.

Adults who consistently break peer pressure patterns tend to rely on internal reference points rather than social ones. Values, long-term goals, and identity act as stabilizers, reducing sensitivity to momentary approval or rejection. When internal criteria are clear, the brain registers less threat from disagreement and less reward from conformity. The pressure weakens because the expected payoff shrinks.

Importantly, resisting peer pressure does not eliminate social consequences—it reframes them. Some social ties loosen, others strengthen, and new alignments form around shared principles rather than shared compliance. From a neurological standpoint, this represents a shift from short-term reward optimization to long-term coherence. The brain adapts, and what once felt uncomfortable becomes neutral.

Peer pressure does not disappear in adulthood. What changes is whether it operates silently or consciously. When its mechanisms are understood, it loses its leverage—and behavior becomes a choice rather than a reflex.

Reference List

University of Texas at Dallas. (2024, March 8). Peer pressure susceptibility lasts into adulthood. *ScienceDaily*. Retrieved December 29, 2025 fromwww.sciencedaily.com/releases/2024/03/240306150631.htm

Morris, H., Larsen, J., Catterall, E. *et al.* Peer pressure and alcohol consumption in adults living in the UK: a systematic qualitative review. *BMC Public Health* 20, 1014 (2020). https://doi.org/10.1186/s12889-020-09060-2

Chapter 9:Techniques for Staying Sober

Sobriety is maintained in the mundane, not the dramatic. It's shaped by routines, environments, and the quiet decisions made every day. People who stay sober don't rely on motivation; they reduce temptation, automate good choices, and design their lives to work with human behavior. Consistency, not intensity, is what breaks alcohol's grip.

The Daily Mechanics of Staying Sober

Lasting sobriety is the accumulation of hundreds of small decisions that quietly reinforce each other. Most of these choices happen in ordinary moments—what you do after work, how you structure your evenings, what you expose your mind to when no one is watching. Strength comes from reducing how often willpower is needed in the first place.

Early recovery demands tighter control because your system hasn't recalibrated yet. In the first few months, the brain is still adapting to the absence of alcohol, which is why cravings, restlessness, and distorted thinking feel so intense. This is where structure matters. You don't rely on optimism—you rely on design. You change routines, limit exposure to high-risk environments, keep your schedule predictable, and stay in regular contact with people who reinforce your decision to stay sober. These actions aren't signs of weakness. They're practical safeguards while your nervous system relearns balance.

Maintenance looks different. As cravings lose intensity, the work shifts from avoidance to construction. The question becomes less about what to stay away from and more about what you are actively building. Long-term sobriety is stabilized by meaning, accountability, and mental health hygiene—things like consistent sleep, honest relationships, purposeful work, and habits that regulate stress before it spills over. When your days are filled with routines that support clarity and self-respect, alcohol stops feeling like a solution and starts feeling irrelevant. That shift—not sheer discipline—is what sustains sobriety over time.

Daily repetition builds resilience the same way physical training does—through accumulation, not intensity. Most protective habits are small and unimpressive on their own: setting an intention in the morning, checking in with someone midday, pausing instead of reacting when stress spikes, reviewing the day before sleep. None of these actions prevent relapse by themselves. What matters is the pattern they create. Over time, these repeated behaviors form a buffer that slows impulsive decisions and creates space between urge and action. That pause is often the difference between relapse and restraint—texting someone before answering an old invitation, or driving a familiar route that bypasses the liquor store without forcing a conscious battle.

To make this reliable, sobriety needs checkpoints built into the day. A short morning commitment sets direction. A simple plan for predictable stress keeps surprises from becoming excuses. A midday self-check catches drift before it turns into damage. An evening review reinforces what worked and exposes weak spots without judgment. Weekly planning—meetings, meals, backup options—reduces reliance on motivation and replaces it with structure. These tools aren't about positive thinking; they're about staying oriented when judgment is tired, emotions are loud, and old habits are looking for an opening.

Routines That Close the Loop

Morning routines work because they intercept behavior before habit takes over. The first hour after waking is when your brain is most suggestible—patterns aren't locked in yet. What you do here sets the tone for how decisions get made later.

A short, daily meditation functions as a circuit breaker. Sitting still for fifteen minutes, focusing on the breath, and letting thoughts pass without engagement trains one skill: noticing urges without obeying them. That pause weakens automatic reactions— the same reactions that once led straight to drinking.

Immediately after, intention setting turns awareness into direction. Three minutes is enough. Ask one concrete question: "What strength will I need today?" The goal isn't inspiration; it's alignment. You're deciding early how you'll respond when pressure shows up.

Journaling comes next because it forces clarity before pressure shows up. When thoughts stay unspoken, they loop and escalate. Writing interrupts that cycle. Five minutes is enough. The goal isn't insight—it's rehearsal.

Simple prompts work best: "What would a successful day look like? How will I handle stress if it hits?" Answering these questions in writing trains the brain to run through scenarios calmly instead of reacting on impulse. Grammar doesn't matter. Polishing doesn't matter. What matters is putting decisions on paper before triggers arrive.

Journaling turns vague intentions into concrete decisions. When plans are written down, they stop floating and start carrying weight. This shift—from thinking about change to acting on it—strengthens follow-through and reduces impulsive choices.

Physical movement comes next because it resets the body before the day gains momentum. Even a short burst—seven minutes of burpees, jumping jacks, or squats—raises energy and lowers baseline anxiety. Slower options work too: stretching or simple yoga wakes the muscles and releases tension. What matters is consistency. Moving your body at the same time each day ties sobriety to action, not motivation. Intensity is optional. Repetition is not.

Gratitude closes the morning loop. Writing down three things you appreciate—even small ones—trains your mind to focus on what's going right instead of what's wrong. Some people reinforce this by sharing one item daily with a trusted partner, adding light accountability. Over time, this practice changes what the mind scans for. When your baseline state includes small everyday positives, alcohol loses its appeal as an emotional shortcut. It stops looking like a solution because the problem feels smaller."

Evenings are the danger zone. Energy is low, structure is gone, and old patterns try to reassert themselves. That's why the night needs just as much intention as the morning. Cutting off screens 30 minutes before bed lowers stimulation and prevents the mental drift that feeds impulsive decisions. Replace scrolling with low-input activities—reading, calm music, light stretching—that signal the day is closing. Keeping a consistent bedtime allows the body to recover, while removing alcohol-related reminders helps cut temptation. Laying out tomorrow's wellness items—meditation cushion, journal, sneakers—acts as a promise to oneself. Reflection comes next. A short journal check-in is enough: one thing that worked, one moment that tested you, and one adjustment for tomorrow. This isn't self-analysis. It's course correction. A five-minute breathing exercise releases built-up tension from the day, and a last written intention closes off the need to ruminate. You end the day conscious, not reactive, and you go to sleep with the next move already decided.

Grounding Techniques

5-4-3-2-1 Sensory Exercise

Sit or stand, plant both feet on the floor.

Silently list 5 things you see—any objects or colors nearby.

Notice 4 things you can feel—clothing, air on your skin, the floor under your feet.

Listen for 3 sounds—inside or outside.

Notice 2 smells—strong or faint.

Name 1 thing you can taste or recall a favorite taste. Doing this redirects focus away from craving and into the present. Use it at work, in a crowd, or alone at home. Each round takes about 2 minutes.

Physical Grounding: Feet-to-Floor

Stand or sit upright.

Press your feet flat into the floor.

Pay close attention to how the ground feels under you.

Push gently, tighten leg muscles, breathe slowly. This gives a sense of steadiness and helps break the tunnel vision of urges. Use anytime, especially if feeling lightheaded or 'floaty'. Repeat as needed.

Temperature Change

Grab an ice cube, splash cold water on your face, or run your hands under a cold tap. Notice the chill and how your body reacts.

Set the object down or dry off, inhale deeply. A temperature jolt resets the body's alarm system, making urges easier to manage. Use when anxiety spikes or distraction fails.

Breathing Methods

Square Breathing

Inhale through the nose 4 counts.

Hold breath 4 counts.

Exhale through mouth 4 counts.

Hold empty 4 counts.

Repeat for 2-3 minutes.

Steadies your heartbeat, calms panic, boosts clear thinking. Try first thing in the morning, after a trigger, or before sleep. Square tracing with your finger can help anchor the count.

Belly Breathing With Hand Guide

Place one hand on your belly and one on your chest.

Breathe in through your nose; feel your belly rise.

Exhale slowly through pursed lips.

Practice for two minutes to ease tense muscles, send calm signals throughout your body, and create a mental pause. Great during traffic, arguments, or when facing a craving.

Counting Breath Patterns

Pick a comfortable number (3, 4, or 5).

Inhale for the count, exhale for the same count.

Find a rhythm that feels natural.

Counting gives your mind a job and keeps attention away from urges. Use sitting, standing, or lying down, any time throughout the day.

Distraction Strategies

Physical Activities

Walk briskly for five minutes around the block.

Drop to the floor and do pushups, crunches, or stretches.

Quick movement shakes up stuck energy, gives your mind a pattern to follow, and can create a sense of accomplishment.

Mental Tasks

Try a fast word association game—list foods, animals, or cities.

Tackle a quick math problem in your head or on paper.

Anything that grabs your full attention can deflate a rising craving. Do these waiting in line or while sitting at a desk.

Productive Redirection

Wash dishes or fold laundry for a few minutes.

Start a mini creative task—write a list for a story, sketch a doodle, or organize a shelf.

Building a sense of purpose distracts from urges and leaves you with something positive in the end.

Practice each of these exercises once a day outside stressful moments. Doing them when relaxed means your brain starts reaching for them naturally when under pressure. Over time, they work hand in hand with your routines, building a solid base for the mindset work ahead and making every day's recovery efforts add up to bigger change.

Sobriety Affirmations for Trigger Moments

Words shape beliefs most strongly under stress. In trigger moments, the brain defaults to familiar scripts tied to relief and habit. Short, intentional statements can interrupt that loop and redirect attention toward values and self-control. These affirmations are designed for moments when urges spike. Use them as written or adapt them so they feel natural and credible to you.

- "I choose a clear mind and a healthy body today."

- "I can tolerate discomfort without escaping it."

- "I protect my boundaries with honesty and self-respect."

- "Sober connection is real connection."

- "Progress counts, even on difficult days."

Write them on paper, save them on your phone, or pair them with routines like breathing or grounding exercises. The goal isn't to convince yourself everything is fine—it's to remind your brain of the direction you've already chosen.

<u>Sober Success Rehearsal</u>

This exercise builds confidence for social situations where alcohol is present by mentally rehearsing success before it happens.

Sit somewhere quiet for about ten minutes. Picture yourself arriving at a social gathering feeling calm and grounded. See yourself smiling, moving comfortably through the space, and choosing a non-alcoholic drink without hesitation. Imagine starting conversations, laughing, and enjoying the moment without needing alcohol to participate.

If someone offers you a drink, visualize yourself responding clearly and confidently with a simple "No, thank you." Notice the sense of pride and control that follows. End the rehearsal by sitting with that feeling of accomplishment for a few seconds.

Practicing this mental run-through lowers anxiety, increases self-trust, and makes sober choices feel familiar rather than stressful. Repeating it before challenging events helps your brain treat success as the default outcome.

<u>Tracking Wins and Building Momentum</u>

Keeping track of your journey reinforces your commitment and offers proof you can look back on. Some find success with a calendar—mark each sober day with a bright color. Others use a detailed mood journal, capturing triggers and victories. Apps tailored for privacy, such as sobriety trackers with password protection, help keep accountability personal and consistent.

Micro-goals—like attending three support meetings or going one week without a drink—make progress manageable. Treat yourself to meaningful rewards when you achieve these benchmarks: a new book, a nature walk, or time with supportive friends.

Accountability Partners

Working with the right accountability partner multiplies your motivation. Choose someone reliable who supports your goals. Set expectations early. Try using phrases like:

"Would you be open to checking in with me once a week?"

"I'd like to talk when I'm struggling—are you comfortable with that?"

"If I cross a boundary, can you remind me of what I set out to do?"

In group support meetings, shared stories create a chain reaction of hope and insight. Group wisdom offers lessons you might not see alone. Protect your own needs with simple boundary scripts: "Thank you for your advice. I'll let you know what works for me."

Designing a Supportive Environment

Finding practical ways to support sobriety starts with reshaping your physical environment so healthy choices require less effort than old habits. Once progress is being tracked and routines are forming, your surroundings either reinforce those changes or quietly work against them. Small, deliberate adjustments in your home reduce friction, limit exposure to triggers, and support consistency without relying on willpower.

A home assessment kicks things off—walk through each room and write down every object or area linked to your former drinking patterns. Be honest and detail-oriented, with a list that might include wine glasses gathering dust, a bottle opener tucked in a kitchen drawer, cocktail recipe books, or that favorite chair where you sipped in the evenings. Entertainment areas often hide triggers—think of a specific lamp, artwork, or playlist once paired with alcohol-centered gatherings. Even subtle cues like leftover bar tools or coaster collections might evoke old routines.

Once the inventory is complete, decide what stays, what gets removed, and what can be repurposed. Some items may need to leave entirely—donating glassware, recycling bar tools, or storing alcohol-related objects out of sight. Others can be reassigned. A former bar cart can become a tea or coffee station. Shelves that once held bottles can display books, plants, or meaningful objects tied to your sober identity. The goal is not to erase the past but to reduce automatic cues that pull attention toward old habits.

Next, build visual and physical cues that reinforce your current goals. Place reminders of progress where they naturally catch your eye: a calendar marking sober days, a journal left open on a desk, or workout shoes by the door. Stock easy alternatives—sparkling water, herbal teas, non-alcoholic drinks—so that when stress or boredom hits, the healthier option is already within reach. Convenience matters more than motivation in these moments.

Finally, pay attention to high-risk time windows. If evenings were once your drinking zone, redesign that part of the day and the space around it. Change lighting, rearrange furniture, or introduce a new ritual like reading, stretching, or walking after dinner. These changes signal to the brain that the old loop has been interrupted. Over time, the environment stops triggering cravings and starts supporting stability, without requiring constant self-control.

Reference List

Kitzinger, R. H., Gardner, J. A., Moran, M., Celkos, C., Fasano, N., Linares, E., Muthee, J., & Royzner, G. (2023, January). *Habits and Routines of Adults in Early Recovery From Substance Use Disorder: Clinical and Research Implications From a Mixed Methodology Exploratory Study*. Substance Abuse: Research and Treatment. https://doi.org/10.1177/11782218231153843

Chapter 10:Building a Support System

Some people don't face hard moments alone. When stress hits or resolve weakens, there's someone who notices, checks in, or quietly keeps them grounded. Others move through the same situations isolated, relying entirely on willpower. The difference isn't strength or discipline—it's whether support is built into their life or left to chance.

Sobriety exposes this gap fast. When alcohol is removed, the social structures around it often disappear too. What remains—or doesn't—reveals how much influence other people have on your decisions, emotions, and follow-through. A support system isn't about constant encouragement or motivation. It's about reducing friction when things get difficult and increasing stability when self-control isn't enough.

Why Support Matters

Recovery outcomes are not evenly distributed. People with strong social connections are far more likely to stay sober than those relying on isolation and willpower alone. Longitudinal research shows that individuals with reliable support networks are roughly twice as likely to remain sober one year after treatment. In tracked recovery samples, about 64% of those with consistent support maintained sobriety at one year, compared to only 34% of those attempting recovery alone.

Support doesn't just improve sobriety rates; it changes how recovery unfolds over time. People with regular peer or group support experience fewer relapses and recover faster after setbacks than those with limited connection. In studies of mutual-aid group participation, individuals engaged in consistent group support increased their total sober days by approximately 27% over twelve months, while those without regular check-ins showed little to no improvement. After a lapse, access to trusted support reduces discouragement and shortens the time to re-engagement with recovery behaviors. Even brief contact—a phone call or message —during periods of craving can interrupt relapse trajectories.

Support also plays a measurable role in mental health during recovery. People who feel socially connected report lower anxiety, fewer depressive symptoms, and greater optimism over time. Research on online, peer-led support groups shows that both individuals in recovery and their family members gain confidence in managing life challenges after participation—even without in-person contact. Participants reported stronger coping skills, access to practical tools, and reduced feelings of isolation. The numbers back this up: people involved in peer recovery programs report more confidence in handling tough situations and greater overall life satisfaction.

Connection also supports recovery in less visible but equally critical ways. Shame—one of addiction's strongest relapse drivers —loses power when experiences are shared with someone who understands. Peers, trusted friends, or supportive family members can reframe setbacks as part of the process rather than personal failure. Simply knowing there is someone to contact during high-risk moments reduces acute stress, while belonging to a group that values honesty reinforces long-term commitment.

These benefits extend beyond emotional relief into daily, practical support. Peer supporters often help solve real-world problems, such as arranging transportation to counseling or planning ways to avoid high-risk situations. In a real-world recovery program, participants reported that having access to peer support in their own community and on their own terms was decisive when confronting everyday temptations and ingrained habits. This combination of shared experience and hands-on assistance makes recovery plans easier to follow and sustain.

Accountability is another powerful benefit of connection. People who participate in group meetings, scheduled check-ins, or regular conversations with a recovery partner are more likely to follow through on commitments because their progress is visible to someone else. Accountability shifts recovery from a private struggle to a shared responsibility. Seeing others maintain sobriety also strengthens belief in long-term success by offering real, living proof that change is achievable.

Understanding the Support Around You

Support during recovery often comes from ordinary connections: family, friends, loved ones, neighbors, coworkers. Informal support might be a check-in call, a ride to an appointment, or someone listening when you need to talk. Sometimes it's quieter —a text reminding you you're not alone, or a sibling respecting your boundaries when you skip the bar this year. Strong support shows up without judgment and celebrates progress, no matter how small. You hear it in simple words: "I've got you," or, "I'm here when you're ready."

Yet, not all support from loved ones feels helpful. Well-meaning family may push advice or cross boundaries, making you feel exposed or guilty. Friends who refuse to respect your limits, like insisting you join them at places or events that feel risky, can pull you off track. Healthy boundaries in informal support matter —choosing what you share, being clear about what is and isn't okay, saying no when offers cross a line, and knowing when to take a break from certain conversations. An example of strong informal support looks like a friend noticing you're struggling and asking, "Do you want advice, or do you want me to just listen?" Unhealthy informal support, in contrast, shows up as a loved one sharing your story without your consent or making you feel like a burden.

Peer support groups bring together people with shared lived experience. A mutual-help group is typically led by peers—folks who 'get it' because they've been there. Twelve-step groups like Alcoholics Anonymous (AA) often follow a fixed format of sharing, reading literature, and encouraging sponsorship, while SMART Recovery groups use open discussions and practical activities based on cognitive and behavioral ideas. Group meetings may be in-person or online, lasting about an hour, with everyone given the space to introduce themselves, share—if they want—or listen and learn. Expectations in these settings include maintaining confidentiality, mutual respect, and attendance without pressure.

Mapping Your Support Network

Building a support network takes intention and a bit of structure, starting with an honest look at who's around you and how you interact with them. Begin this journey by mapping out your circle and exploring ways to reach out for help, both from people you already know and from unexpected sources.

Start by listing every relationship in your life on a sheet of paper. Friends, family, co-workers, neighbors, past teachers, group leaders—no one is too obvious or too peripheral to consider. Once you have your list, assign each person a rating: supportive, neutral, or risky. Supportive individuals respect your boundaries, show care, and have acted helpfully in the past. Neutrals neither help nor hinder. Risky relationships could encourage old habits or challenge your recovery goals.

Write down the best way to reach each person (call, text, email, social media, in-person), their typical availability, and the communication method they respond to best. Record their contact details so it's easy to reach out in a moment of need. For everyone rated as supportive or neutral, jot down one practical way they might help: offer company, drive you to appointments, or just listen. For those considered risky, note what boundaries you need or if pauses in contact are wise.

Before moving forward, run through these questions for each relationship:

Does this person respect my limits and privacy?

How did they react last time I needed help?

Are they themselves in a good spot, with a healthy attitude toward alcohol or substances?

When they commit, do they follow through?

Can I trust them with sensitive information?

Being honest here builds a realistic, personalized support network, not just an ideal one.

Hidden Allies Discovery

You might have untapped support right around you. People from everyday activities can become unexpected allies. Make a list of your regular groups—work teams, hobby circles, religious or community gatherings. See if any members stand out as kind, trustworthy, or supportive. This could include workplace mentors who check in with how you're doing, a neighbor who's always up for a chat, someone in your book club, or a friend of the family who's overcome tough times themselves. Extended family, even if not in touch regularly, may surprise you; sometimes a cousin or aunt can step in as a steady contact. Former teachers, classmates, or supervisors can be solid too, since they might offer encouragement with a bit of distance from daily life.

Script Development for Asking Support

Having the right words ready makes difficult asks much easier. Start your script by thanking the person for their friendship or relationship. Share your request clearly, keep it short, and explain how their help would make a difference. Offer options—maybe they can't meet every week, but a monthly check-in is doable. End with gratitude, no matter their answer.

Here are script templates you can adapt:

Alcohol-Free Socializing

"I really enjoy spending time together and trust your support. I'm working on building healthier routines and would appreciate if we could do things that don't involve alcohol. This would help me stay on track and feel more comfortable. Would you be willing to plan some sober activities with me? Of course, only if it works for you."

Check-In Calls

"Your friendship means a lot. I've found regular check-ins help me, and I'm wondering if you'd be open to having a quick call once a week. It would give me something to look forward to and keep me motivated. Let me know if that's possible."

Emergency Contact

"I value our connection and trust you a lot. I'm putting together a list of emergency contacts. Would you be okay with being one? I'd hope not to need help often, but just knowing you're someone I could call would bring peace of mind."

Boundaries

"I care about you and our relationship. I'm working on some personal changes, and for now I'd like to avoid being around alcohol when we're together. It would help me stay steady, and I'd still love to see you. Thanks for understanding."

Emotional Support

"I really appreciate how you listen. Sometimes I go through tough moments, and simply talking helps. Would you be willing to hear me out when things get hard? Anything you offer is enough."

Communication Do's and Don'ts

Do:

Say clearly what you need and when

Be thankful for any help offered

Give the other person a real choice and honor their answer

Propose simple actions, not vague "be there for me" statements

Don't:

Demand support or use guilt to convince someone

Push someone to take charge of your processes

Leave things unclear ("Maybe you could help sometime…")

Support Circle Blueprint

Make a list of three concrete tasks to complete this week for your support network. Pick two people to ask for help and write a script for each. Choose specific days to reach out and jot down how you'll thank them, whether or not they say yes. By building this blueprint, you move from thinking about support to making it real, setting up the foundation for more structured accountability relationships.

Choosing Accountability That Works

When you map out your support system, seeing names on a list helps you notice who shows up and how. Turning these names into active accountability partners means thinking about the strengths and boundaries of each relationship. Maybe your cousin is great with early-morning texts, while your friend from work likes phone calls after dinner. The key is asking people for help in ways they feel good about and making your needs clear. You could say, "Would you be open to texting with me at 9am each day just to check in?" or "Can I call you on Sunday afternoons to talk through my week?" It's honest and simple, and lets both people know what to expect.

Setting up accountability doesn't have to be complicated. It helps to make the system easy to follow, with routines that can stick. For people who like structure, daily check-ins might work best. For others, using an app to log wins or struggles feels more natural. You can agree to send a message every morning that says, "Checking in—ready to take on today." You might set a standing phone call every Sunday at 4pm. Spell out what happens if you miss a check-in: "If I forget our check-in, will you reach out and send me a reminder?" or "Let's talk about any time check-ins don't happen to see what could help." This helps lower shame and stress, making the process about support, not punishment.

Accountability can feel heavy if the tone is all about calling out mistakes. Keeping it positive is about focusing on what's working rather than only what's missing. Share wins, no matter how small. Give your accountability partner a script for how they can support you: "It really helps if you ask me what felt hardest today, or what made me smile." This can keep check-ins friendly and human, not just tasks to complete. Let your partner share too —accountability is stronger when it flows both ways.

If you're looking for group support, choosing the right one matters. Ask yourself does the group leader explain how things work? Do members greet new people with warmth, or are newcomers left to guess what's going on? Watch for practical tips you can use at home. Check if the group welcomes questions about harm reduction, 12-step, SMART Recovery, or other ways to get better—nobody should be shamed for choosing what works for them. If you hear lots of "this is the only way" or sense shame-based messaging, those are red flags. You deserve a space where you feel safe to share wins and struggles without harsh judgment.

The same rules apply at home. Family plays a unique role in accountability, often making things trickier. Sometimes loved ones mean well but end up enabling, like covering for missed work, making excuses, or taking over your responsibilities. This can block growth even as it feels like help. Healthy support boosts your sense of autonomy and respect. If someone keeps stepping in, you can set a boundary with simple language: "I appreciate your concern, but I need to handle this my way." You might also ask for something specific: "It would help me most if you could offer encouragement, not solutions." Imagine a parent dropping by unannounced to check on you; a calm response could be, "I'd prefer you call first next time. I need some space, and I'll reach out if I'm struggling." Or, if a partner wants to control your recovery: "I need to take responsibility for these steps myself, but I'd love your support if I hit a roadblock." Saying it out loud takes practice, and you can rehearse with a trusted friend or in a support group.

For some, family support isn't possible or feels unsafe. In those cases, it's okay to look elsewhere—many find second families in peer support groups, or with trusted friends and mentors. Family members might also need help of their own, through therapy or groups like Al-Anon, Nar-Anon, or parent groups, especially if they're struggling to let go or feeling isolated. These options create a bridge to professional help, showing both you and your loved ones that recovery often needs outside support. Online support and telehealth can make these connections easier to access, letting more people be part of your team without barriers of distance or schedules. Every step you take toward clear accountability and healthy boundaries makes your support system sturdier and brings a little more peace to everyone involved.

Reference List

Engaging Family and Others in Recovery | Research Corner | IRIS. (2024). IRIS . https://www.iris.ssw.umaryland.edu/rc-family-recovery

Scannell, C. (2021, January). *Voices of hope: Substance use peer support in a system of care*. Substance Abuse: Research and Treatment. https://doi.org/10.1177/11782218211050360

Zemore, S. E., Lui, C. K., Mericle, A. A., Li, L., Martinez, P., & Timko, C. (2025, July 1). *Second-wave mutual-help groups: Examining effectiveness for individuals with alcohol use disorders in the longitudinal, U.S. national PAL Study cohorts*. International Journal of Drug Policy; Elsevier BV. https://doi.org/10.1016/j.drugpo.2025.104921

Chapter 11: The Science of Alcohol Recovery

Why does quitting alcohol feel like such an uphill battle? Why do urges hit so hard, even when you've decided to change? And why do some people achieve lasting recovery while others struggle repeatedly? These questions go beyond willpower—they're about what's happening in your brain. Understanding this is key to real change. Let's explore how biology, psychology, and proven treatments work together to make recovery possible.

The Path to Recovery

Recovery science is a field that explains how biology, psychology, and evidence-based methods work together to help people move beyond addiction. The core idea is simple: with the right tools, anyone can change. Recovery starts by understanding how alcohol, drugs, or unhealthy patterns affect the brain. For example, behavioral therapy uses exercises that help people practice new ways of responding to stress or cravings, actually changing the strength and direction of brain circuits over time. When someone learns what triggers an urge to use and develops new coping skills, the brain slowly builds new pathways, like forming a different trail through a dense forest. These changes are not just theoretical —they are visible in brain scans, and they show up in increased success rates for people seeking lasting recovery.

At the heart of recovery science is the concept that the brain is not fixed. Brain chemistry changes with addictive behavior, but the brain can also heal and adapt. Take neural plasticity as an example. The brain works like a network of trails in a park. When a person repeats the same action, such as turning to alcohol after a stressful day, the pathway becomes worn-in, making it the easiest route to take. Over time, these routines become automatic. But when someone makes intentional choices—like calling a friend instead of drinking, or pausing to breathe when stressed—they slowly create new trails. These new connections get stronger with practice. Eventually, these healthier habits can become just as automatic as the old ones used to be over time.

Science also sheds light on why recovery can feel like an uphill battle at times. Alcohol and other drugs disrupt neurotransmitter balance, which means motivation, pleasure, judgment, and self-control become harder. Medication-assisted recovery offers extra help in these moments by addressing the brain's chemistry. For instance, medications can reduce cravings or block the "reward" signal when using, making it easier to build new habits without falling into old traps. These treatments boost success rates, helping people stay on track, and are a powerful option when used with therapy.

Medication is just one piece of the puzzle. Evidence-based approaches to recovery come in several forms, each with a clear goal. Behavioral therapies, such as cognitive-behavioral therapy (CBT), teach practical skills: how to spot and interrupt triggers, how to replace risky behaviors, and how to manage stress before it leads to relapse. Motivational approaches, such as motivational interviewing, tap into a person's own reasons for change, building commitment step by step. People set goals that matter to them and map out small, achievable steps. Medication-assisted treatment, or MAT, supports the physical side of withdrawal and craving, so people don't have to rely on sheer willpower alone.

These treatments are not just theories. Brain scans show real differences before and after recovery. For example, research finds that people who practice behavioral skills can "rewire" parts of the brain linked to impulse control and planning. Success rates tell the same story: people who get evidence-based treatment are more likely to reach long-term recovery, with studies showing improved outcomes after one year, three years, or even longer. The combination of therapy, medication, and support raises the chance of success—something that would not be possible if addiction were only a matter of willpower.

Learning about recovery science also reduces shame. People see that addiction is a pattern the brain can pick up, not a personal failing. When someone understands that their struggle is part of a brain process, they are more likely to ask for help, join treatment, and stick with changes. Families and communities who understand these facts offer better support, and people beginning recovery feel less alone.

Science does more than explain; it provides a practical roadmap. By showing how habits are formed and changed, highlighting the success of different therapies, and giving hope based on long-term data, recovery science encourages people to take the next step. Treatments are chosen based on what works, not on old ideas or guesswork, and every new study adds more proof that recovery is possible.

With a clear understanding of brain chemistry and why the brain develops habits, the path is open for a closer look at the brain's reward system and neural pathways. This deeper look helps explain why certain triggers and rewards shape behavior and shows how targeted therapies turn scientific insights into practical change.

Psychological Principles Behind Addiction

Patterns of behavior in alcohol use disorder often begin with familiar situations and emotions. Picture coming home after a long day, tense from deadlines or difficult coworkers. That stressed, exhausted feeling can trigger an almost automatic stop at a bar—sometimes without conscious planning. This sequence of trigger, urge, and response is not a failure of willpower. Over time, alcohol conditions the brain's reward system to link specific cues—such as work stress or social gatherings—with drinking routines.

Once this pattern is established, it unfolds quickly: a feeling sparks a thought, the thought leads to action, and the brain briefly registers relief or pleasure. The same routine can repeat across many settings—at a Friday office party, a family dinner, or alone after a breakup.

Cognitive distortions are thought patterns that twist reality and keep drinking cycles going. You might hear yourself think, "Just one drink won't hurt," even after promising to stop—this is minimization, a way of downplaying risk and consequences. After a setback, thoughts like "I'll never be able to quit" reflect all-or-nothing thinking. Other common distortions include catastrophizing ("If I relapse, everything is ruined") and overgeneralization ("Every time I try to quit, I fail"). These mental shortcuts create a false sense of certainty. Over time, as the brain's reward system adapts, alcohol can start to feel like the only solution in certain moments.

Common Cognitive Distortions and Examples

Minimization: "I only drink on weekends, it's not a big deal."

Catastrophizing: "If I slip once, there's no hope for me."

All-or-nothing thinking: "I failed to stay sober at the party, so I'm doomed."

Personalization: "If my friends see me not drinking, they'll reject me."

Discounting positives: "Sure, I've cut back, but that doesn't count."

These thoughts seem automatic, but they're habits shaped by the brain's changed chemistry. Learning to spot and question them is the first step away from old patterns.

Mindset and motivation play a big role in change. Alcohol may feel necessary in some situations, but examining your thoughts and beliefs can open up new options. Take a moment to ask yourself:

"When do I feel most tempted to drink?"

"What do I tell myself before I decide to have a drink?"

"What do I want my relationship with alcohol to look like a year from now?"

Notice which situations feel hardest to handle without alcohol and which feel easier. These differences highlight where planning, support, or new coping skills will matter most.

Pattern Recognition Exercise

Notice triggering situations (work stress, social events, loneliness)

Document the automatic thought ("I need a drink to relax")

Identify the behavior that follows (stopping at a bar, pouring a drink at home)

Record how you felt during and after (relief, guilt, tiredness)

Look across several situations for repeated patterns

Cognitive Distortion Checker

Write down your thoughts about drinking, especially in high-risk moments

Check them against the list of distortions above

Ask yourself: Is this thought totally true? Is there another way to see it?

Try writing a more balanced thought ("One slip doesn't erase all my efforts")

Read your new thoughts out loud when tempted, practicing the new pattern

Learning these strategies taps into your brain's neuroplasticity—the ability to form new connections even after years of ingrained habits. Each time you notice a trigger, challenge a thought, or choose a different response, you strengthen new neural pathways. This doesn't erase the struggle, but it shows that thoughts and behaviors tied to alcohol are both identifiable and changeable.

Catching yourself in these loops and practicing new ways of thinking lays the groundwork for lasting change. Relapse can happen during learning, but each attempt to recognize patterns or adjust thinking builds skill and resilience. With the right knowledge and support, the brain continues to adapt, making healthier patterns more accessible over time.

Evidence-Based Treatment Approaches

Cognitive Behavioral Therapy (CBT) is one of the most widely studied approaches for changing drinking patterns. It's based on the idea that thoughts, feelings, and behaviors are linked—and that shifting one can affect the others. Treatment often begins by identifying triggers and high-risk situations, such as loneliness after work or passing a familiar bar.

Clients may keep a daily log of drinking episodes, noting the situation, thoughts, and emotions beforehand. This functional analysis breaks behavior into steps, revealing patterns that usually run on autopilot. Once visible, CBT focuses on practical skills to interrupt them.

Those skills might include practicing how to refuse a drink, challenging thoughts like "I deserve this," or learning ways to handle anger or social anxiety. For example, someone who believes they can't enjoy parties without alcohol might test that belief by attending sober and noticing what actually happens. Planning for high-risk events—holidays, stress, social pressure—is another focus. Research shows structured CBT programs can reduce relapse risk by 30–40%, with lasting benefits for those who stick with the process.

Motivational Interviewing (MI) takes a different approach. Instead of challenging behaviors and thoughts directly, MI creates a space where people can explore their own reasons for change. The four main principles—expressing empathy, developing discrepancy, rolling with resistance, and supporting self-efficacy—form the basis of every MI session.

For example, an MI counselor listens carefully, reflects back the person's words, and shows understanding without judgment. In one session, the person might say, "I don't see why I need to stop drinking. It's just what I do with my friends." The counselor could respond, "It sounds like socializing with your friends is really important to you." This simple phrase, grounded in empathy, helps the person feel understood and open up. That sense of safety is what allows honest self-reflection to begin.

Developing discrepancy means gently helping people see the gap between current habits and future goals. A counselor might say, "You mentioned wanting to feel healthier and be more reliable for your family. How does drinking fit into those goals?" This question helps people weigh their priorities and often leads to moments of insight.

Medication support offers another recovery tool. Doctors may suggest medications such as naltrexone, acamprosate, or disulfiram for people seeking extra help, especially if cravings and relapse risk remain high. Naltrexone works by blocking the pleasurable buzz alcohol gives, which can reduce the urge to drink. Acamprosate helps with withdrawal symptoms by balancing brain chemistry. Disulfiram, on the other hand, causes uncomfortable reactions (like nausea) if a person drinks, which serves as a strong deterrent.

Medications are often started after detox and combined with therapy. Naltrexone and acamprosate usually start to show benefits in a few weeks and may be taken for several months or longer depending on progress. Research shows that people who use these medications alongside counseling are less likely to relapse, with success rates jumping by up to 25–30% compared to those who go without any medication.

No single treatment fits everyone, but these proven strategies —CBT, MI, and medication support—work together to replace old patterns with new, healthier ones. Regular check-ins measure progress. Goals often shift from daily drinking reduction to celebrating first sober milestones and building routines that support long-term health. Therapy, encouragement, and practical planning all help make lasting change possible.

Tracking Progress & Common Misconceptions

Making daily progress visible is possible with simple tools like a dedicated recovery journal. Each morning or evening, pick up a notebook or open a digital document and jot down three prompts: "How am I feeling?", "What triggered cravings or slips today?", and "What worked for me today?"

Tracking patterns over time—whether mentally, through brief notes, or during therapy—helps people notice links between mood, routines, and high-risk moments. Looking back on these patterns often shows which strategies reduce cravings and which situations need extra support. This kind of feedback makes approaches like CBT more responsive and personal.

Some people use recovery apps as a lightweight way to notice trends rather than to "manage" recovery. Seeing changes in mood, time sober, or stress levels over weeks can highlight common trigger windows, such as weekends or demanding workdays. When used thoughtfully, these tools can complement therapy by reinforcing awareness—not replacing human support.

Support groups add a social dimension to progress and accountability. Many people find that regularly hearing others' experiences—and sharing their own—helps turn abstract insights into lived change. Conversations often focus on small wins, moments of temptation, or setbacks and what they revealed. Talking through these experiences reinforces skills learned in CBT or motivational interviewing, while also reducing isolation. Over time, this shared reflection strengthens motivation and makes recovery feel less like a private struggle and more like a collective effort.

Measuring progress can feel abstract without concrete signs. Often, change appears first in everyday functioning rather than emotions. Sleep becomes more regular, with fewer nighttime interruptions and more consistent wake times. Energy levels stabilize, making mornings easier. Work attendance improves, and sick days or missed responsibilities decrease. Relationships also offer clues—conversations feel calmer, family interactions are more positive, and new social connections start to form. These objective shifts often emerge before people fully recognize the emotional benefits of recovery.

Overcoming Barriers in Alcohol Recovery

Culture adds another layer. In families or communities where drinking anchors social life, recovery often requires more than saying no. Bringing non-alcoholic options or asking friends for quiet support can make a difference, especially where alcohol is deeply ingrained.

Recovery approaches varied widely. Peer support groups offered structure and accountability, with participants attending meetings weekly or more, in person or online. Some groups focused on shared experiences—new parents, veterans, or members of specific cultural communities. For many, this peer model provided consistent encouragement and reliable check-ins.

Choosing the most effective recovery method often depended on personal circumstances. Young adults juggling school schedules gravitated toward online group support rather than in-person meetings. People in rural areas relied on teletherapy or phone counseling to avoid long commutes. Single parents adapted routines or used flexible online resources to fit around work and childcare. Seniors tended to prefer smaller, age-specific groups where their experiences were understood and respected.

Money and geography shaped choices and sometimes limited options. Participants in larger cities had access to diverse programs but sometimes struggled with costs. Those in small towns reported fewer choices but often experienced more consistent, close-knit support. Time was a precious resource, with many describing the need to "squeeze in" meetings, therapy, or exercise around jobs and family demands. For most, finding the right balance between what was available and what they could realistically commit to made all the difference.

Pitfalls surfaced in the form of relapse triggers, usually noted in personal diaries. Birthdays and holidays topped the list. One participant described two solid weeks of progress until facing a friend's milestone celebration. Surrounded by laughter and champagne, she hesitated. Her strategy: carry a glass of sparkling water with lime, keeping her hands busy so offers felt easier to turn down. Still, the night ended with her accepting a drink out of discomfort. The next day, she wrote about her guilt but also about a plan: schedule a check-in call with her group leader before the next event and rehearse her responses to common pressure lines.

Isolation had its own daily signals. One man in a small apartment felt alone each evening. At first, he filled the time with TV, but boredom led to temptation. He switched things up by signing up for short online courses, using those hours as both a distraction and a skill-builder. Progress was visible: after tracking his evenings in a journal, the urge window shrank from three hours to just forty-five minutes over two weeks, turning the weakest time of day into a manageable one.

Reference List

Hammoud, N., & Jimenez-Shahed, J. (2019, February). *Chronic Neurologic Effects of Alcohol*. Clinics in Liver Disease. https://doi.org/10.1016/j.cld.2018.09.010

Noble, J. M., & Weimer, L. H. (2014, June). *Neurologic Complications of Alcoholism*. CONTINUUM: Lifelong Learning in Neurology. https://doi.org/10.1212/01.con.0000450970.99322.84

Pados, E., Kovács, A., Kiss, D., Kassai, S., Kapitány-Fövény, M., Dávid, F., Karsai, S., Terebessy, A., Demetrovics, Z., Griffiths, M. D., & Rácz, J. (2020, January 3). *Voices of Temporary Sobriety – A Diary Study of an Alcohol-Free Month in Hungary*. Substance Use & Misuse. https://doi.org/10.1080/10826084.2019.1705861

Chapter 12: Where to Find Help

Most people wait too long to get help because they misunderstand what help actually is. It isn't only rehab, group confession, or labeling yourself as anything. It's access to structure, information, and accountability when self-control alone stops working. The moment alcohol starts taking more time, energy, or mental space than you want to give it, outside support becomes a rational option. This chapter lays out what those options are and how they differ, so help can be used deliberately rather than emotionally.

Digital Tools for Support

These apps focus on tracking your alcohol intake, logging your progress, and building accountability. They make it easier to notice patterns, reinforce consistency, and stay on top of your recovery journey.

Sober Grid

Sober Grid is a social network for people in recovery that lets you track your drinking and connect with peers anywhere in the world. It helps by giving real-time accountability and support, which reduces the mental strain of self-monitoring alone. Using it is simple: log each drink or milestone, and check in with the community when cravings hit to get encouragement or advice.

I Am Sober

I Am Sober is a daily tracker that visualizes your progress with streaks, reminders, and motivational prompts. It helps the brain by reinforcing consistent routines and rewarding small wins, which strengthens decision-making and mental clarity. To use it effectively, start each day by logging your sober intent and mark milestones as you go — the visual streaks make your progress tangible.

Loosid

Loosid combines alcohol tracking with lifestyle and social features, including local sober events and community forums. It reduces impulsive drinking by giving structured routines and social cues, which also lowers stress and supports overall health. Simply set up your profile, track your days, and explore local events or connect with peers when you need accountability.

Nomo

Nomo is a minimalist sobriety timer that tracks your alcohol-free days and lets you share progress with friends. It helps by turning abstract goals into measurable results, reinforcing consistency and self-discipline. Use it by starting a timer each day you remain sober and checking your dashboard to see streaks and progress over time.

SoberTool

SoberTool uses behavioral psychology to prevent relapse, sending motivational messages, reminders, and small exercises when cravings occur. It helps by training your brain to respond to triggers without drinking, reducing stress-related gut and mental strain. Simply open the app when you feel a craving or at daily check-ins to reinforce positive behaviors.

Next, these apps focus on meditation and mindfulness, helping calm the mind, manage stress, and reduce cravings—the mental triggers that often lead to drinking.

Headspace

Headspace is a guided meditation app with sessions for stress relief, focus, and sleep. It helps by calming the nervous system, lowering cortisol, and reducing cravings triggered by stress or anxiety. To use it, pick a short daily session—starting with 5–10 minutes is enough—and follow the guided voice to train your mind to pause before reacting to urges.

Calm

Calm offers meditation, breathing exercises, and sleep stories designed to relax the mind and body. Regular use reduces stress, improves sleep quality, and stabilizes mood, which can indirectly support gut health and cognitive clarity. Simply choose a session that fits your day—morning for focus, evening for winding down—and stick to a consistent schedule.

Insight Timer

Insight Timer gives access to thousands of free guided meditations and music tracks. It works by helping you create a personalized mindfulness routine, reinforcing emotional regulation and lowering impulsivity related to drinking. Use it by selecting a short daily meditation or a background timer for mindful breathing, even while doing other tasks.

10% Happier

This app emphasizes practical, science-backed mindfulness techniques aimed at reducing stress and improving self-awareness. It helps the brain recognize cravings and respond without reacting, which strengthens self-control circuits. Start by following the beginner courses and practice short daily sessions, then gradually increase session length as comfort grows.

Breethe

Breethe combines meditation, sleep aids, and life coaching to manage stress and emotional triggers. Regular use supports the body's recovery from alcohol-induced stress and promotes emotional stability. To use it, choose a session that matches your current need—stress relief, motivation, or sleep—and integrate it into a daily routine for consistency.

**These apps use music, soundscapes, and binaural beats to
calm the nervous system, improve focus, and reduce stress—
the mental triggers that often lead to drinking.**

Brain.fm

Brain.fm uses AI-generated music designed to improve focus,
relaxation, and sleep. Listening helps regulate brainwaves,
lowering stress and reducing impulsive urges linked to alcohol.
Use it by selecting a session for focus or relaxation and listening
through headphones for 15–30 minutes, ideally daily.

Endel

Endel creates personalized soundscapes based on your
environment, time of day, and heart rate. These soundscapes
reduce cortisol and calm the mind, helping the brain resist triggers
for alcohol. Simply start a session in the morning to focus or at
night to unwind—consistency strengthens the effect.

Binaural Beats Therapy

This app delivers audio tracks with carefully tuned frequencies
that influence brainwave activity. Regular use helps improve
mood, sleep, and mental clarity, indirectly supporting recovery by
reducing stress-driven cravings. Listen daily for 10–20 minutes,
ideally in a quiet space with headphones.

Relax Melodies

Relax Melodies allows you to mix sounds and music for
meditation, sleep, or stress relief. It helps lower anxiety and
improves sleep quality, giving your body a better environment to
recover from alcohol-related stress. Use it by creating a
personalized mix each night before bed or during short relaxation
breaks.

Insight Timer – Music Tracks

Beyond meditation, Insight Timer offers music and ambient tracks specifically designed for stress reduction and focus. These tracks help the brain maintain calm and reduce triggers for drinking. Listen for 10–15 minutes during breaks or meditation sessions to reinforce emotional regulation.

These next tools use psychology, reframing exercises, and behavior change techniques to reduce cravings, strengthen self-awareness, and build mental resilience against drinking triggers.

Reframe

Reframe is built around short daily exercises that help you notice automatic thoughts and consciously shift your mindset. It's like having a coach that prompts you to question cravings and rewire unhelpful thinking patterns. Use it daily for 5–10 minutes to catch triggers early and challenge them before you act — simple but effective practice that strengthens cognitive control.

Youper

Youper blends AI-guided conversations with psychological techniques (CBT, mindfulness, reframing) to help users unpack emotions that drive cravings. You talk to the app like a coach, get prompts to rethink your urges, and track mood over time. Use it when you feel a craving or at set check-ins — consistency builds emotional regulation and reduces stress-driven drinking.

Wysa

Wysa uses conversational AI and evidence-based tools to coach you through difficult emotions and triggers. It's mainly for mood and anxiety, but those are often at the root of cravings. Use Wysa to journal feelings, complete bite-sized exercises, or do thought reframing when stress spikes — the goal is to strengthen your default response to triggers.

Moodfit

Moodfit isn't specifically for addiction, but it uses daily check-ins, mental exercises, and habit tracking that mirror NLP principles. The app helps you map how mood, sleep, stress, and behavior interact — so you see patterns instead of acting on them reflexively. Use Moodfit each morning to set intentions and each evening to reflect, building predictability in your responses.

Stories That Inspire Recovery

Books can be a powerful companion in recovery. They provide insight into the challenges of addiction, illustrate real-life experiences, and show the strategies others have used to regain control. Reading the right book can inspire change, offer practical guidance, and give perspective on the mental, emotional, and social aspects of quitting or reducing alcohol.

These three books are highly rated on Amazon for their personal journeys of addiction and recovery, offering lessons, insight, and inspiration for anyone working to change their relationship with alcohol.

Drinking: A Love Story — Caroline Knapp

A candid memoir by journalist Caroline Knapp about her long, complicated relationship with alcohol — from early attraction to obsession and its impact on her life. Knapp's writing pulls no punches: she describes the psychological pull of drinking and how it quietly consumed her life before she recognized the pattern and began to change it. This book is helpful because it feels like listening to someone you know talk honestly about how and why they arrived at addiction and what the first steps toward change looked like for them.

Blackout — Sarah Hepola

In *Blackout*, Sarah Hepola shares her own experiences with heavy drinking, including the frightening realities of blackout drinking — episodes she couldn't remember — and how that shaped her sense of self and relationships. Hepola combines tough honesty with insight about how our culture treats alcohol, why blackouts happen, and what it takes to reclaim control. This book resonates because it blends personal story with reflection on the mental and emotional cost of alcohol, making readers think differently about their own patterns.

Asylum (Alcoholic Takes the Cure) — William Seabrook

An older classic but one of the earliest confessional memoirs of alcoholism, Seabrook chronicles his institutionalization for alcoholism in the 1930s. It's honest, raw, and haunting in the way only firsthand experience can be. Though written decades ago, it still conveys how devastating and consuming alcohol addiction can be and what recovery looks like from the inside out. For readers who want perspective on the lived experience of addiction itself, this book delivers powerful insight.

Here are three workbooks that can support your recovery journey.

The Alcohol Experiment Workbook — Annie Grace

This companion to *The Alcohol Experiment* guides you through 30 days of reflection, goal-setting, and habit tracking. It helps you examine your drinking patterns, recognize triggers, and take small, structured steps toward change. Use it daily to track progress and apply insights in real time.

This Naked Mind Workbook — Annie Grace

The workbook version of *This Naked Mind* provides exercises that reinforce the book's principles, helping you challenge beliefs about alcohol, notice thought patterns, and create a plan for lasting change. Regular use strengthens awareness and builds practical skills for managing cravings and social pressures.

The Mindful Drinking Journal — Rosamund Dean

A combination of journaling prompts and exercises designed to encourage mindful reflection on alcohol use. It helps users track drinking habits, emotions, and triggers while encouraging mindful choices. Daily entries promote self-awareness, reduce impulsivity, and support gradual, intentional change.

These books provide a research-based look at alcohol and addiction, explaining how it affects the brain, body, and behavior, and offering evidence-backed insights.

The Science of Addiction — Carlton K. Erickson

This book breaks down the neurobiology behind addiction, explaining how brain reward systems, genetics, and neural pathways are involved in compulsive alcohol and drug use. It frames addiction not as a moral failing but as a biological process, helping readers understand the *physical mechanisms that drive cravings and dependency.* This is useful for anyone trying to make sense of why willpower alone often isn't enough.

Healing the Addicted Brain — Harold C. Urschel, M.D.

Written by an addiction psychiatrist, this guide uses neuroscience and clinical research to explain how addiction alters brain chemistry, why cravings persist, and what evidence-based strategies help the brain recover. It goes beyond willpower to give readers a scientific framework for retraining the brain and reducing relapse, grounding recovery in biological reality rather than myth.

Proof: The Science of Booze — Adam Rogers

This book explores how alcohol works in the body and brain from a scientific perspective, from fermentation chemistry to physiological effects like hangovers and long-term impacts. While not a recovery manual per se, it gives readers a deep, research-oriented look at how alcohol interacts with neural systems, cognition, and bodily functions — helping you understand the science behind what you're quitting or moderating.

Online Resources

The right websites can be a real turning point in recovery, offering immediate access to expert guidance, supportive communities, and practical tools. Whether you're trying to understand cravings, track progress, or connect with people who truly get it, these resources make help feel accessible rather than distant.

The sites listed below offer practical guidance, peer support, and tools designed to help manage cravings and stay grounded in recovery.

SMART Recovery (smartrecovery.org)

SMART Recovery is an evidence-based program that helps people manage addictive behaviors, including alcohol. It provides tools, worksheets, and online meetings to teach practical skills for coping with cravings, making better decisions, and building a life free from alcohol. Use it by exploring their free resources, joining online meetings, or downloading their worksheets to track progress and practice recovery techniques daily.

Alcoholics Anonymous (aa.org)

AA is the classic 12-step program with a global network of in-person and online meetings. It offers peer support, guidance, and structured steps to help individuals maintain sobriety. You can use the website to find meetings near you, learn about the 12-step process, and access online literature that helps reinforce recovery principles.

Rethinking Drinking (rethinkingdrinking.niaaa.nih.gov)

This site, from the National Institute on Alcohol Abuse and Alcoholism, provides science-based guidance on drinking patterns, risks, and strategies for cutting back or quitting. It offers self-assessment tools, interactive guides, and research-backed advice. Use it to understand your drinking habits, see personalized feedback, and plan practical steps toward healthier choices.

Soberistas (soberistas.com)

Soberistas is an online community for people looking to reduce or quit alcohol, with a focus on peer support and shared experiences. It helps by connecting you with people who understand the challenges of drinking, offering discussion forums, articles, and encouragement. Use it by joining the community, participating in conversations, and drawing inspiration from real-life stories and advice.

These online communities and forums provide ongoing support, peer advice, and real-life experiences, giving you a place to connect, share, and learn from others.

r/stopdrinking (Reddit)

Large active subreddit dedicated to people quitting or reducing alcohol. Users post personal experiences, daily check-ins, and advice. It helps by providing peer accountability, encouragement, and real-world tips. You can use it by following threads, posting updates, or reading archived posts for insight.

Sober Recovery Forum (soberrecovery.com)

A long-standing forum where people share experiences, ask questions, and get guidance from peers and moderators. It covers alcohol and other addictions. Helpful because it's structured into topics and searchable, letting you find advice relevant to your exact situation. Check in regularly and contribute to threads to build connection and accountability.

Facebook – Sober Support Groups

Many Facebook groups focus on sobriety, moderation, and peer support (e.g., "Soberistas Community," "Sober and Thriving"). They're private, moderated, and active daily. These help by giving a mix of motivation, advice, and social interaction. Join a group, introduce yourself, and engage with posts to maintain a sense of community and accountability.

InTheRooms (intherooms.com)

An online recovery community with discussion forums, chat rooms, and virtual meetings. It's built to last and caters specifically to alcohol and addiction recovery. Use it by joining forums, participating in meetings, and reading discussions to stay connected with others in recovery around the clock.

Alcohol-related charities can provide crucial support, guidance, and resources to help you navigate recovery, and once you've made progress, they also offer ways to give back.

Facing Addiction (facingaddiction.org)

Facing Addiction provides education, advocacy, and resources for people affected by substance use. It helps by connecting you with treatment programs, support groups, and practical guides for recovery. Use it by exploring their informational guides, joining webinars, or accessing referral tools to find local help. Once you're progressing in your own recovery, you can engage with their advocacy efforts to support others.

Shatterproof (shatterproof.org)

Shatterproof aims to end addiction's devastation through education, support, and research. It helps readers by offering evidence-based information, treatment locators, and programs to guide recovery decisions. Use it by reviewing their resources, finding treatment centers, or participating in awareness campaigns. Later, you can contribute or volunteer to strengthen the recovery community.

The Betty Ford Center (bettyfordcenter.org)

A nonprofit treatment center founded by Betty Ford, it provides counseling, programs, and support for people struggling with alcohol and substance use. It helps by offering structured treatment, educational resources, and peer support, whether in-person or online. You can use their online materials to learn strategies for managing cravings and building a healthy routine. As you recover, you may choose to support the center's programs through donations or volunteer work.

Addiction Policy Forum (addictionpolicy.org)

This nonprofit focuses on education, advocacy, and connecting individuals to evidence-based addiction resources. It helps by giving access to treatment options, webinars, and research-backed guidance on recovery. Use it to learn about available programs, connect with specialists, and explore tools for managing alcohol use. Once established in recovery, you can participate in advocacy initiatives to help others navigate the system.

While online resources and apps are helpful, nothing replaces the power of face-to-face connection. Local support groups and meetings give you accountability, guidance, and a sense of community you can't get alone. They let you share experiences, learn from others who understand your challenges, and build relationships that reinforce your recovery journey. Even a single regular meeting can make a significant difference in staying on track and feeling supported.

For many, Christian churches are a familiar place to find in-person support groups and recovery programs. If your faith is different, you can explore the following communities to find support for your journey — simply search online to locate the nearest center. These centers offer connection, guidance, and structured programs that support sobriety.

Buddhism

Buddhist temples and meditation centers provide classes, mindfulness workshops, and peer groups focused on mental clarity and emotional balance. Regular practice of meditation and mindful living can reduce cravings, improve focus, and strengthen self-control. To find a nearby center, visit www.buddhanet.info and use their "Find a Temple or Center" tool. Participating in group meditation sessions or mindfulness workshops can reinforce consistency in recovery.

Hinduism

Hindu temples often host community gatherings, wellness programs, and cultural events that emphasize discipline, self-reflection, and ethical living. Some centers also provide counseling or peer support for life challenges, including addiction. You can find a nice local Hindu temple or program through www.hinduamerican.org/resources/temples.

Islam / Muslim

Mosques and Islamic centers offer community counseling, educational workshops, and peer support programs. Engaging with these centers can help you develop structure, accountability, and a support network while learning stress management and ethical decision-making practices from a faith perspective. Locate your nearest mosque or center at https://www.islamicfinder.org and consider joining study circles, counseling sessions, or support groups offered there.

Judaism / Jewish

Synagogues and Jewish community centers provide educational programs, social support, and counseling services. These communities emphasize connection, shared values, and structured activities that can reinforce positive habits and resilience during recovery. Visit https://www.jewishfederations.org to find centers near you. Participating in group events or counseling sessions helps build accountability and a sense of belonging.

Sikhism

Gurdwaras are known for strong community ties, volunteer programs, and support networks. They emphasize service, discipline, and mindfulness, which can help you develop habits that support recovery. To locate a gurdwara near you, check https://www.sikhnet.com/gurdwaras. Joining community events or volunteering can reinforce routine, connection, and purpose, all of which strengthen sobriety.

If you're not interested in religious-based programs but still want face-to-face guidance, accountability, and community support, there are several secular in-person groups that can help you on your recovery journey. Many of these programs operate across multiple English-speaking countries.

Alcoholics Anonymous Again (AA)

Although AA has already been mentioned earlier in this book, it is included again here because it is the largest and most widely available recovery support organization in the world. AA operates in more than 180 countries and offers both in-person and online meetings, making it one of the easiest ways to access support regardless of location. While AA includes spiritual principles, many groups focus primarily on shared experience, peer support, accountability, and long-term consistency in recovery.

Women for Sobriety (WFS)

Women for Sobriety is a peer-support organization designed specifically for women seeking recovery from alcohol dependence. The program emphasizes emotional growth, self-esteem, and personal responsibility through structured peer support. Women for Sobriety operates primarily in the United States and also offers online meetings, making it accessible to women in other English-speaking countries.

Secular Organizations for Sobriety (SOS)

Secular Organizations for Sobriety is a recovery network that emphasizes personal responsibility, rational decision-making, and long-term self-control. The program focuses on practical thinking, accountability, and peer support to help individuals maintain sobriety. SOS groups operate in the United States, Canada, the United Kingdom, Australia, and also offer online meetings for broader access.

LifeRing Secular Recovery

LifeRing is a peer-led recovery organization that takes a secular, self-empowering approach to sobriety. Meetings focus on strengthening sober thinking, sharing practical strategies, and supporting personal growth through mutual encouragement. LifeRing operates in the United States, Canada, the United Kingdom, Australia, and New Zealand, with both in-person and online meetings available.

Moderation Management (MM)

Moderation Management is designed for individuals who want to reduce or better control their drinking rather than immediately commit to full abstinence. The program uses behavioral tools, goal-setting, and self-monitoring to help participants reshape their relationship with alcohol. Moderation Management is most active in the United States and Canada, with online options available for participants in other countries.

Not everyone connects with structured recovery programs or formal organizations. Many people benefit from smaller, community-led groups created by individuals who share similar goals and experiences. These options offer flexibility, local connection, and support that feels more natural and approachable.

Meetup.com

Meetup allows people to create and join local groups centered around shared interests, including sobriety, alcohol-free living, and recovery support. These groups may focus on discussion, accountability, or sober social activities. Searching for terms like "sober," "alcohol-free," or "recovery" in your city can help you find groups that match your comfort level.

Facebook Groups

Facebook hosts many active sobriety and recovery groups, including location-based and interest-specific communities. These groups offer ongoing conversation, shared experiences, and peer support without requiring formal participation. You can join private or public groups and engage at your own pace.

Local Community Centers

Community centers, libraries, and wellness spaces often host peer-led support groups related to recovery and mental health. These gatherings are usually informal and accessible, making them a good option for in-person connection without a structured program. Checking local calendars or bulletin boards can uncover nearby opportunities.

University or Workplace Wellness Groups

Some universities and workplaces provide alcohol-free or recovery-friendly support groups through wellness programs. These groups offer peer support in familiar environments and can help reinforce accountability within daily routines.

Sober Social Communities

Sober social groups focus on building connection through alcohol-free activities such as fitness, outdoor events, or casual meetups. These communities help people rebuild a social life without alcohol and reduce isolation during recovery.

<u>*Government and Public Health Support*</u>

Many governments offer free or low-cost alcohol support through public health systems. These services often include counseling referrals, community programs, helplines, and medically supervised care. While names vary by country, they're usually accessed through national or regional health agencies.

In the United States and Canada, support is commonly available through public health departments, community clinics, and national helplines. In the United Kingdom, Australia, and New Zealand, similar services operate through national health systems and local councils. A simple search for "alcohol support services" or "substance use help" along with your city or country can lead you to official resources.

These options are especially helpful if you need professional guidance, medical oversight, or referrals to local programs. Even if you prefer peer-led or community-based support, government resources can help point you in the right direction. With these tools available, you can build accountability and take meaningful steps toward lasting change by choosing what fits you best.

Chapter 13:Life After Sobriety

Life after sobriety isn't a finish line—it's a series of daily choices that gradually shape a different life. This chapter explores how routines, small decisions, and mindful strategies turn early efforts into lasting change. Living without alcohol unfolds through repeated actions—skipping a drink at a work event, stocking foods you actually enjoy, planning for lonely Friday nights—that quietly add up over time.

Each day offers a new chance to decide how you'll respond to stress, face challenges, and care for yourself. These choices may seem small in isolation, but practiced consistently, they reshape your reality.

A big part of sustaining sobriety is how you see yourself. There's a difference between telling yourself "just don't drink today" and actually believing "I'm not someone who drinks." The first is about willpower, which can feel exhausting, especially when you're tired, anxious, or out with friends. The second involves a deep shift in your sense of identity. Seeing yourself as a non-drinker transforms choices from constant struggles into natural extensions of who you are. Drinking loses its place in your life because it no longer fits the story you tell yourself.

Managing Emotions and Connections

Recognizing and naming emotions gives you power over them. Pause during the day when you notice strong feelings—frustration, boredom, anxiety, or excitement—and ask yourself, "What exactly am I feeling?" Jot a quick note or use a mental check-in. Over time, you'll start spotting patterns and understanding which situations consistently trigger certain emotions.

When emotions threaten to overwhelm, bring yourself back to the present with a sensory grounding check-in. Instead of the morning exercise, keep it flexible: notice one or two things you can see, one sound, one sensation in your body, and one thing you can imagine tasting or smelling. The goal isn't a rigid routine—it's a quick, portable tool to interrupt spiraling thoughts and respond intentionally rather than react automatically.

Some emotions demand attention from a professional. If anger becomes uncontrollable, sadness lingers for weeks, sleep and appetite change without improving, or you withdraw from activities and people you like, consider therapy or support group meetings. Listen to feedback from close friends or family. If loved ones express concern about mood swings, or you feel unsafe with your own thoughts, reach out for help right away.

Navigating parties, dinners, and social events sober can feel awkward. Prepared scripts smooth the path. When someone offers you a drink, try, "I'm good with water, thanks," or "I don't drink, but I'm happy to raise a toast with this soda." Keep your response friendly and relaxed. Another option: "No thanks, I've switched to non-alcoholic drinks—tell me about your summer vacation." Changing the topic invites connection without focusing on your choice.

Bringing your own drinks demonstrates confidence and self-care. Carry flavored sparkling water, lemonade, or tea in a reusable bottle or thermos. Ask the host ahead of time if you can pop your drink in the fridge or bring a small cooler. This small step can stop last-minute stress and put you in control of what's in your glass.

Planning your exit gives you freedom. Scope out the layout when you arrive—find a quiet spot for a breather, and decide how long you want to stay. If you need to leave early, use a phrase like "I've got an early day tomorrow," or "I'm catching up on rest these days." Choose honesty if you're comfortable, or keep it simple if that fits better for you.

Supportive relationships flourish with clear, honest communication. For partners, try: "When you have a glass of wine, I feel left out. Can we plan an activity together that doesn't involve alcohol?" With a friend or family member: "I'm focused on sobriety, and I appreciate your support." Setting boundaries helps everyone involved. If others try to pressure you, respond with: "I understand you want me to join in, but I'm choosing what's best for me." Say it with warmth but stand firm.

Look for ways to connect that don't revolve around drinking. Host a board game night, join a book club, take a walk in the park, or try a new recipe with friends. Celebrate milestones by visiting a favorite coffee shop, catching a movie, or taking a small trip. These moments build pleasure and pride without risking your progress.

Success grows from practical action. Julian felt anxious about a friend's wedding but prepared responses and brought his own drinks. He left when he started feeling overwhelmed and woke up grateful for his choices. Lara faced her old drinking buddy at a weekend picnic, saying, "I'm doing things differently now, and I'd still love to see you." They connected over a shared meal, and Lara realized their friendship could shift and grow.

Daily emotional check-ins, quick regulation techniques, and supportive social strategies work together to help you catch warning signs early. By paying attention to your feelings in the moment and building confidence in social settings, you learn to protect your progress and keep your recovery strong.

Protecting Your Progress

Long-term sobriety relies less on willpower and more on noticing trouble early and responding quickly. Temptation rarely arrives out of nowhere—it builds through subtle shifts in mood, thinking, and routine. Recognizing these early signals gives you a chance to act before a close call becomes a setback. Slips and near-misses are common, especially early on, and each one offers information about how to protect your recovery more effectively.

Often, the first warning signs are mental. You may start thinking you no longer need meetings, therapy, or check-ins. Isolation can creep in, even when support once helped. Romanticizing past drinking is another early signal.

Behavioral changes tend to follow. Maybe you stop reaching out, cancel meetings, or quietly drift from your support system. Physical cues matter too: restless sleep, skipped meals, reliance on sugar, or feeling constantly run-down. Emotional shifts often appear alongside these—irritability, unexplained sadness, or rising anxiety. These signals aren't failures; they're prompts to use the tools you've built.

One skill that makes a huge difference is urge-surfing. When a craving hits, start by noticing it without judging yourself. Rate the craving from 1 to 10, just to get a sense of its strength. Take a moment to check in with your body—are your shoulders tense? Is your heart racing? Take a slow breath in, then release it. Set a timer for five minutes. Instead of fighting the urge, watch it come and go like a wave. With practice, you'll see that cravings do rise and fall. When time is up, rate the craving again. Most people notice it's dropped, even if just a little. That's a win.

Having a personalized prevention plan will give you a sense of control. Start by listing your personal triggers. Who or what makes you want to drink? Is it certain places, or particular moods? Write them down. Next, identify your early warning signs— maybe sleep problems, feeling edgy, or skipping support activities. Make a list of who you'll contact in tough moments— your sponsor, a best friend, a counselor. Jot down your most reliable coping strategies for hard moments, whether it's taking a walk, texting a friend, or using urge-surfing. Remove anything in your space that might tempt you, like bottles, hidden cans, or even barware. Stock healthy snacks or drinks in the fridge. Decide on a quick daily check-in routine—maybe an evening journal note—to spot trouble early and stay ahead.

A crisis can come up fast, so it helps to have words ready. If you need to reach out to a friend, you might say, "I'm feeling off today and really need someone to talk to. Can you stay on the phone with me for a few minutes?" If someone offers you a drink, a simple, "No thanks, I don't drink anymore" works. If you need to be firmer, try, "I'm working on my health. Alcohol isn't part of my life now." When cravings feel intense, quiet self-talk goes a long way: "This feeling will pass. I've gotten through worse. I am not my craving."

Real changes in your environment can help prevent surprises. Remove anything linked to drinking from your space. Play music that makes you feel calm. Keep fizzy water, tea, or favorite snacks within reach. Scope out exits and have plans for leaving situations that feel risky. Every time you use these skills—urge-surfing, reaching out, making a smart swap in your space—you're not just avoiding relapse, you're proving to yourself that you're building something solid. Each day you use what you've learned, you add another brick to your foundation. This is what makes your achievements real and worth celebrating in your recovery story.

Recognizing Progress and Staying Motivated

The first week free from alcohol often feels like climbing a tall hill, but that first Friday night without drinking is a victory all its own. One idea is to mark it with something bright and simple, such as treating yourself to your favorite meal, buying a plant, or taking a day trip to a park. People often celebrate with close friends or family who support their progress. That positive feeling carries you through the early cravings. Tools for relapse prevention like urge surfing, tracking triggers, and reaching out to support groups act as sturdy handrails during these moments.

After a month, changes start to show up in the mirror and in how you greet each day. Stories from clinical research show that sleep, which is often jagged at first, gets better and deeper after 2 to 3 weeks. People mention waking up clear instead of groggy, with energy that lasts past noon. Cravings are easier to handle, and negative moods soften as your body's natural rhythms come back. This is a natural place for a new milestone celebration: maybe a picnic, a day at a museum, or a new hobby. Tracking improvements like "I slept 7 hours straight," or "I needed less coffee," is a real boost.

At six months, major benefits show up in physical health. You may notice smoother skin, weight loss of 5-10 pounds, and a happier digestive system. Blood pressure starts to normalize, and liver enzyme levels often improve — something routine checkups can confirm. Headaches and heartburn fade away. One way to honor this milestone is to buy yourself new clothes or gear for a sport—something that shows off your healthier body and spirit. Some choose to run a 5k or join walking groups, using their new energy to build social ties.

Reaching a year of sobriety is a major transformation. Often you find yourself looking at the world with a clearer head; decision-making feels less pressured. Mental clarity means you remember things more easily, and anxiety is less likely to hijack your day. People commonly mention stronger job performance, new promotions, or starting classes they never would have taken before. For many, this milestone means gathering loved ones for a dinner or a trip, marking the anniversary with something memorable and alcohol-free.

Reference List

Lorman, W. J. (2013, September). *Maintaining Sobriety and Recovery.* Nursing Clinics of North America. https://doi.org/10.1016/j.cnur.2013.04.005

McKay, J. R. (2021). *Impact of Continuing Care on Recovery from Substance Use Disorder.* Alcohol Research: Current Reviews. https://doi.org/10.35946/arcr.v41.1.01

Support Recovery: It's a Marathon, Not a Sprint | National Institute on Alcohol Abuse and Alcoholism (NIAAA). (n.d.). Www.niaaa.nih.gov. https://www.niaaa.nih.gov/health-professionals-communities/core-resource-on-alcohol/support-recovery-its-marathon-not-sprint

Conclusion

So what happens now, after you close this book? This is where action counts. It's time to choose at least one new habit or strategy from these pages and put it into practice today. Start small, but start. Maybe it's swapping your evening drink for a walk, reaching out to a trusted friend, journaling about why you want to stay sober, or joining an online group for accountability. Each small win builds momentum, helping you to trust yourself and see real progress over time.

I want to leave you with a personal reflection, because the path toward sobriety is deeply personal for me, too. When I decided to make a change, I didn't do it all at once or get every step "right." Some days were miserable, others full of hope. What got me through wasn't superhuman willpower, but a combination of practical support, honest self-reflection, and the willingness to try again, even after setbacks. With time, I began to notice subtle shifts: more laughter with friends, clearer mornings, fewer regrets. Eventually, those little moments turned into something bigger—a genuine sense of freedom I hadn't felt in years.

Thank you for trusting yourself enough to begin, and for allowing this book to be part of your process. May your next chapter be filled with clarity, strength, and joy. Your future self is already grateful for the choices you make today.

www.ingramcontent.com/pod-product-compliance
Lightning Source LLC
Chambersburg PA
CBHW022106050726
47591CB00002B/691